PELVIC PAIN

A MUSCULOSKELETAL
APPROACH FOR TREATMENT

Peter Dornan AM DIP PHTY, FASMF

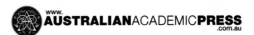
www.
AUSTRALIANACADEMICPRESS
.com.au

First published 2014
Australian Academic Press Group Pty. Ltd.
18 Victor Russell Drive
Samford Valley QLD 4520
Australia
www.australianacademicpress.com.au

National Library of Australia Cataloguing-in-Publication entry

Creator:	Dornan, Peter, 1943- author.
Title:	Pelvic pain : a musculoskeletal approach for treatment /
	Peter Dornan.
ISBN:	9781922117366 (paperback)
Subjects:	Pelvic pain--Treatment.
	Pain--Treatment.
	Sacroiliac joint.
	Musculoskeletal system--Diseases--Physical therapy.

Dewey Number: 617.55

Publisher & Editor: Stephen May

Design & Typesetting: Australian Academic Press

Illustration support: Karen Mounsey-Smith and Maria Biaggini

Cover image: ©iStock.com/7activestudio

Printing: Lightning Source

Contents

It is the mark of an educated mind to rest satisfied with the degree of precision which the nature of the subject admits and not to seek exactness where only an approximation is possible.

— Aristotle (Nicomachean Ethics, 1. iii. 4)

Not everything that counts can be counted and not everything that can be counted counts.

— Einstein

This book is dedicated to my youngest grandson, Archer Bruijn.

— Peter Dornan

Acknowledgments

A book of this nature relies heavily on the support of not only members of the medical profession, but also on the many sufferers, survivors and patients who have shared their problems and experiences with me. The collective courage, humility and support by individual members continue to inspire me.

I would particularly like to acknowledge the role of my colleagues from the Centre of Clinical Research Excellence (CCRE) Spine at the University of Queensland, Drs Michel Coppieters, Paul Hodges, Gwen Jull and Ruth Sapsford. I am extremely grateful to Michel, my supervisor and co-author during four years of research at the Centre. I am also extremely grateful to Dr Bruce Mitchell, a Sports and Interventional Pain Physician from Metro Spinal Clinic in Melbourne.

I would particularly like to pay tribute to the role of my friend and urologist, Dr Les Thompson, for his insight and consistent encouragement and direction over the last ten years with this project. I am indebted also to the many other urologists, radiologists, other specialists, doctors and physiotherapists who have assisted me to further my understanding in this area, particularly special members of the Continence and Women's Health Special Group of the Australian Physiotherapy Association.

A special accolade also goes to my dedicated Office Manager, Carol Marchant, whose patience and assistance in both typing and compiling the many drafts of this manuscript has been invaluable. In this regard I would also like to thank my publisher, Stephen May, for his always helpful guidance. Special thanks also to Karen and Maria for their work on several of the anatomical drawings and the pudendal nerve map.

I wish also to express my gratitude to the many caring friends and health professionals I have met both internationally and locally, especially through the International Pelvic Pain Society (IPPS) and Professor Thierry Vancaillie's Women's Health and Research Institute at the University of New South Wales.

Finally, I would like to thank my wife, Dimity, for being my continual support system and my tireless cheer squad leader when problems seemed insurmountable.

Peter Dornan AM

About the Author

For 48 years, Peter Dornan has been a physiotherapist in the fields of sports medicine and manipulative therapy, working with many international sporting teams, including the Australian national rugby union team, the Australian national rugby league team, the Queensland rugby union team, and the Australian cricket team. For his achievements, he was awarded the Commemorative 2000 Australian Sports Medal. He is also a passionate Men's Health activist. In 1997, Peter created a forum for men and their partners to gain support and be better informed in matters relating to prostate cancer.

Peter has also been freelance writing for many years and has written two books on sporting injuries, one on prostate cancer, (*Conquering Incontinence*) and four military books (*The Silent Men*, an account of the Kokoda Track Campaign, *Nicky Barr — An Australian Air Ace*, *The Last Man Standing*, an account of the Tobruk and El Alamein Campaigns, and *Diving Stations*, an inspiring story of one of the most successful submarine commanders of World War II).

In 2002, Peter was appointed as a Member of the General Division of the Order of Australia (AM).

Peter is married to Dimity Dornan (AO), a Speech Pathologist, who is the Founder and Executive Director of 'Hear and Say', a world-wide charity which teaches deaf babies to speak. They have two adult children, Melissa and Roderick.

Introduction

I have written this book for patients who have a specific variety of pelvic pain — pain or other symptoms related to the pelvis that does not respond to specialist intervention by physicians, urologists, gynaecologists, gastro-enterologists and pain management specialists.

It is also written for health professionals who are interested in pelvic pain. It will be particularly useful for musculoskeletal therapists. If the patient has any of the following conditions, ones that have resisted traditional medical treatment, it is possible they may well have a musculoskeletal cause.

- Pain (or altered sensations) in the scrotum, penis, labia, vulva, vagina, perineum and pelvic floor region, anorectal region, low abdomen, bladder or prostate region or groin. These 'altered sensations' may be described as stabbing, numbness, tingling, buzzing, electric, deep ache, burning, lumpy feeling or pinching. Patients may report sensations that their pelvic anatomy is altered or missing, such as feeling that the anus or another object is drawn up inside the bowel. The pain can be triggered either from a sudden physical movement or event relating to pelvic dysfunction or from a heightened sensitivity to palpation. It can also be evoked subtly over a long period of time, such as from extended periods of incorrect sitting.

- Dysuria (painful or difficult urination), irritable bowel and/or irritable bladder syndromes, urge incontinence — faecal or urinary, pain during or after defecation or micturition.

- Sexual and erectile dysfunctions including impotence, persistent arousal and priaplasm (persistent erections). Pain during or after intercourse or ejaculation.

- Changes in skin temperature and/or sensory changes in skin, itchiness, redness in lower abdomen areas, groin, thighs or genitals, often producing intolerance to tight underclothes and certain cloth textures. The scrotum may appear darker, shrink and draw up into the pelvis.

To articulate plausible explanations for persistent pelvic pain, a quick look at the medical literature, text books or 'Dr Google', (as most patients already have done) reveals the answer may well be complicated. Generally, authorities will agree the most consistent cause may be a complex interaction between the gastro-intestinal, genito-urinary, musculoskeletal, nervous and endocrine systems, influenced by socio-cultural factors.

A significant number of patients present under the idiopathic (which means we don't really know), non-infective and non-bacterial classifications. During the diagnostic process, specialist medical attention would have considered such common pelvic pain conditions as interstitial cystitis, prostatitis, vulvodynia, endometriosis, cancers and prolapses, ano-rectal dysfunction, proctalgia fugax, pelvic floor muscle pain syndrome, obturator internus and piriformis syndromes, and neuropathic pain (nerve) syndromes. Specialists will uncover many more not-so-usual conditions. **If any of these potential conditions fail to respond to traditional medical treatment, it should be considered that they may have a musculoskeletal cause.**

Further, various types of pain must be considered — nociceptive (which arises from irritation of peripheral sensory nerves — from fractures, sprains or bruises after a fall, perhaps), visceral (from visceral organs, bladder etc. — a disease, perhaps), functional (movement related) and neuropathic, which is the result of injury or malfunction in the peripheral or central nervous system. I am going to concentrate on this last condition — neuropathic pain.

Neuropathic pain is defined as pain due to nerve damage and/or pain arising as a direct consequence of a lesion or disease affecting the somatosensory system. (Treede et al., 2008). The dominant and particular nerve involved here with the pelvis is the **Pudendal Nerve,** but there are others.

Many pelvic and perineal pains are now categorised as pudendal neuralgia. However, as has already been stated, making such a diagnosis is not easy (and may not be accurate) as many nerves may be involved, from both somatic and autonomic nervous systems. As well, many mechanisms may be involved including damage to other anatomical structures.

In many cases, I contend there may be a musculoskeletal component involved with the cause of these symptoms. Often a clue for this involvement is that the pelvic pain symptoms are regularly associated with a history of low back pain, with or without groin, buttocks and leg symptoms. They are often initiated by sitting or sitting can make them worse. Cycling can be a common cause. More on this later (see pages 16 and 29).

The pudendal nerve supplies each and all of these aforementioned anatomical structures and regions mentioned in the opening paragraphs, and monitors, influences and is associated with their individual functions. The nerve is a key component in providing sensations that range from pleasure to pain. If this nerve is compromised in any way, from its origin to anywhere along its course, it can produce the potential to give rise to any, or a combination of all, of the above symptoms. The diagnosis then is **Pudendal Neuropathy**. There has been some mystery involved with this diagnosis. We should search further.

Pudendal Neuropathy encompasses all diseases of the pudendal nerve and may or may not involve pain. The term **Pudendal Neuralgia** (PN) is a sub heading of Pudendal Neuropathy and describes pain of a severe throbbing or stabbing character in the course of the nerve. Pudendal neuralgia is a neuropathic pain condition involving inflammation and dysfunctional firing of the nerve due to trauma or disease. The nerve can become sensitised and send out heightened signals to the genitals and associated systems.

The term **Pudendal Nerve Entrapment** (PNE) is defined as a focal nerve lesion produced by constriction or mechanical distortion of the nerve anywhere along its course. It can give rise to symptoms of pudendal neuralgia, however, pudendal neuralgia can also result from other causes.

Because the diagnosis PNE implies the nerve may be irrevocably entrapped or caught somewhere, it gives the impression surgery may be the only means of treatment. In reality, only a small minority of patients will have this situation. It is therefore important a clear diagnosis is made. A pudendal nerve block can sometimes ascertain if the pudendal nerve is involved.

In 1990, Labat and others (Labat et al., 1990) stated that anaesthetic pudendal nerve blocks, when used as a diagnostic test, were considered positive if there was total relief of pain when sitting within one hour of infiltration.

More recently it was stated (Labat et al., 2007) that the diagnosis of PNE is essentially clinical. A working party has validated a set of simple diagnostic criteria, called the *Nantes Criteria*. The five essential signs and symptoms are:

1. Pain in the anatomical territory of the pudendal nerve
2. Worsened by sitting
3. The patient is not woken at night by pain
4. No objective sensory loss on clinical examination
5. Positive anaesthetic pudendal nerve block

However, since then, it appears one of the most valid means to diagnose actual entrapment at present is with Magnetic Resonance Neurography, (MRN — a process most simply described as an MRI of a nerve)

Aaron Filler (Filler, 2009), a surgeon from California, has documented four possible different locations of entrapment, by MRN investigation. On a series of 189 patients which were diagnosed with PNE, the four categories he found were:

i   Entrapment exclusively at the level of the piriformis muscle in the sciatic notch only (2%)

ii. Entrapment at the level of the ischial spine and sacrotuberous ligament (5%)

iii. Entrapment in the Alcock (or pudendal) canal on the medial surface of the obturator internus muscle (80%)

iv. Entrapment at the distal branches of the pudendal nerve (13%)

There may now be other methods to make this diagnosis clearer. Professor Thierry Vancaille, a gynaecologist and pain specialist from the University of New South Wales, reported from a 2011 'Pudendalhope' site, that by using dynamic fluoroscopy, a radio-opaque dye is used to localise Alcock's Canal and the infra-piriformis canal. He states he is now developing a technique to combine MRI and the neurography to try and gain a clearer understanding of the anatomy. He also reports that a single injection of a pudendal nerve block results in a substantial improvement in at least 40% of patients.

However, in 2003, Dr Jerome Weiss (Weiss, 2003) reported that Professor Roger Robert, a neurosurgeon in Nantes, France, found in his surgical patients, the source of the entrapment was at the sacrospinous ligament in 58%, and/or the sacrotuberous ligament in 69%, and often included the falciform process of the sacrotuberous ligament in 42%.

The troubling potential prognosis for a compressed or entrapped nerve relates to the pathophysiology involving ischaemia of blood vessels supplying the nerve. Subsequent collagen deposition and fibrosis (scarring) can increase the intraneural pressure and can initiate a self-perpetuating cycle of pain causing neural hypersensitivity.

Importantly, a competent MRN which clears entrapment as a diagnosis can amount to a revelation which is often a liberating moment for these patients. It means they may now be able to confidently search for a more moderate form of treatment than surgery — and be patient when coping with the effects of hypersensitivity.

For the patient, at the initial consultation with their Health Professional, he or she may have considered the end point (or end structure) of that nerve to be the problem. That is, if the patient presents and complains of say, a painful scrotum or vulva, he or she may be diagnosed as having a local condition such as an infected or inflamed testicle (orchialgia) or vulvadynia. The patient may indeed be treated for this diagnosis and perhaps be prescribed antibiotics. This can often give temporary relief as it is known that some antibiotic (anti-bacterial) agents can have a therapeutic anti-inflammatory effect; the precise mechanisms remain to be elucidated. The patient may also be given relieving medications, anti-inflammatories or surgery — in fact, surgical removal of a testicle, or a hysterectomy, (to relieve the pain) is not uncommon. The patient may also be offered other physical interventions, such as injections of Marcaine, steroids, Botox, hyaluronaidase, and intraoperative placement of adhesiolytic agents, typically Seprafilm.

Further, integral with this diagnosis, long-term distress, caused by chronic symptoms, regularly is associated with co-morbidities of depression, anxiety and fear. Couple this with minimally or temporarily effective treatments given by a plethora of physicians and therapists, and the loss of quality of life, can lead to cognitive decline. This situation is then often treated by anti-depressants.

All, or any, of these treatments, including anti-depressants, may temporarily relieve the symptoms. However if the real cause is a compromise of the pudendal nerve, in any of its presentations, the relief may be short-term. (Including for the patient with the removed testicle or hysterectomy).

The patient may then have his/her diagnosis assigned into a different classification — **Chronic Pelvic Pain Syndrome** (CPPS). Chronic pain is defined as daily pain that continues for three months or more. There is a move to change this label to "Persistent Pelvic Pain Syndrome", implying that the word "chronic" may inhibit any treatment program.

I must reinforce there can be several nerves and systems involved with this diagnosis, which I will mention later, but for now, I want to concentrate on the pudendal nerve.

A New Approach

There are obviously many valid ways that the pudendal nerve can be compromised, such as from a disease process, during surgery or from a traumatic sporting or motor vehicle accident. However, clinically, I have observed that many of the above conditions are often associated with pelvic girdle dysfunction involving the sacroiliac joint, which, as I shall explain, can implicate the pudendal nerve.

My argument therefore, is that many forms of persistent pelvic pain may have its origins in pelvic dysfunction which may lead to irritation of structures innervated by the nerve.

Some work has already been done from this angle by physiotherapists. Stephanie Prendergast and Elizabeth Rummer (Prendergast & Rummer, 2006) from San Francisco have charted a number of musculoskeletal impairments which can be associated with pudendal neuragia. They list such conditions as pelvic floor dysfunction, connective tissue restrictions, myofascial trigger points, muscle hypertonicity, altered neurodynamics, sacroiliac joint dysfunction and other structural/biomechanical abnormalities and central sensitisation.

They state that in the case of sacroiliac joint dysfunction, extreme or abnormal joint positions, such as pelvic rotations may result in increased tension on the ligaments through which the pudendal nerve passes. As a result, the ligaments may compress or shear the nerve and lead to inflammation, setting up the painful symptoms.

This concept then will introduce a specific perspective to managing these conditions; a musculoskeletal approach. This different strategy is often a conflicting, difficult and challenging notion to a patient who has had a reinforced belief that something must be wrong at the local end-site, for example, testicle, vulva, prostate, bladder, rectum etc.

As a sports physiotherapist with a strong experience of managing spinal and musculoskeletal conditions what would I know of all of this? Let me breifly explain my involvement.

About eleven years ago, a urologist friend of mine consulted me for treatment of a painful lower back. He sustained it by lifting weights and executing split squat exercises at the gym. It was a routine consultation for me. I was able to deliver a simple diagnosis and prescribe an uncomplicated treatment. I diagnosed him as having sustained a sprained sacroiliac joint where the innominate bone of the pelvis had been forced into extreme posterior rotation on the sacrum (see Figure 8 on page 28). I treated it by selecting an appropriate mobilisation technique and exercises. He phoned the next day to thank me and report that his back pain was gone, and so was his scrotal pain. This was a surprise as I wasn't aware that initially he had scrotal pain. In fact, patients never walk into a physiotherapist at first contact and complain of scrotal pain or any of the aforementioned symptoms — they will rightly go instead to their local doctor.

"What had I done to help with the scrotal pain?" he asked.

My friend confided he had several cases of patients who had presented with scrotal pain which had not responded to treatment — so he would send them to me. One of the first patients had a clinical diagnosis of prostatitis and had been on antibiotics for two years. However, after looking at all his pathology, the urologist found no evidence of any prostatitis or other urological problem. Within two weeks of mobilising and exercise, the symptoms had resolved.

In fact, all the patients responded to this approach. My friend then said "You had better find out what you are doing and why you are getting results". Quick research revealed that the scrotum is supplied predominately by the pudendal nerve (although other nerves can be involved). I also found that the pudendal nerve supplies and controls most of the major organs and systems in the pelvic area. In fact, all of the areas involving the previously cited conditions. That set me off on a serious path of research and discovery.

I went back to university and studied with Michel Coppieters, PhD a physiotherapist who specialises in neural pain. I then revisited the anatomy lab, and with another physiotherapist, Dr Susan Mercer, dissected out the pudendal nerve and followed its course from its origin in the sacrum, at the base of the spine, to where it moves through the pelvis. We then examined its mechanics and relationship with the sacro-iliac joint, the large joint which joins the sacrum to the pelvis. We then looked for possible reasons why damage to this joint could impact on the nerve, then, with this information, I fine-tuned my mobilising techniques and exercise program.

Quite simply, as I shall explain in the coming chapters, and as suggested by Prendergast and Rummer (Prendergast & Rummer, 2006), I considered that if either of the flanking bones of the pelvis, — the innominates (see Figure 8 on page 28) was rotated significantly on the sacrum, (from the result of e.g., injury from sport, work, lying heavily and incorrectly during surgery, or pregnancy or sitting incorrectly), a situation could indeed be set up where the pudendal nerve (and other sacral and lumbar nerves) could be compromised.

It is well accepted now that the nervous system slides and glides as we move. Broadly, as a result of this process, the pudendal nerve could be harmed through several possible mechanisms; compression, stretch, (creating what is known as altered nerve biomechanics) or entrapped between or around other anatomical structures. I proposed that any of these processes could potentially lead to the symptoms detailed at the beginning of this introduction.

A large part of this study was to establish the role that posture, in particular, sitting posture, and lumbar-pelvic mechanics played in causing and managing this condition. Long periods of incorrect sitting were found to be a consistent denominator in the cause, as well as exacerbating the symptoms. This was particularly so amongst workers who sit at computers all day, and with drivers, (taxis, couriers, tractors), and addicted television viewers. Importantly, this research revealed that more nerves than the pudendal nerve may be involved with this scenario.

The final important aspect to address was how to manage and treat hypersensitivity of the nerve. Without correctly identifying the cause of these symptoms, (and therefore addressing and treating the cause) continued repetitive stressing of the nerve, sometimes for years, has the potential to set up debilitating, over-reactive, inappropriate and complex pain cycles, (termed hypersensitivity).

In regards to complex pain cycles, I include several other points for completeness. It is worthwhile mentioning that some therapists consider that the same pudendal neuralgia symptoms could be triggered by viscero-somatic reactions set up by other disease processes in the pelvis. Such conditions as endometriosis, irritable bowel and irritable bladder syndromes, chronic bladder and kidney infections, medical interventions such as hysterectomy and prostatectomy, and conditions which arise from ovarian, uterine, vaginal, vulvi and labial areas, may all set up a painful viscero-somatic reflex. You will note in the diagram of the pudendal nerve map (see Figure 3 on page 15), the pelvic splanchnic nerve (which carries the viscero-somatic nervous system), and the pudendal nerve, both emanate from S2, 3 and 4. It is speculated that this closeness may set up the prospect of "mutual influence" in the nerves.

There is some evidence that suggests that afferent stimuli arising from such a visceral disorder (of any of the above mentioned conditions), through a process known as 'viscerosomatic convergence' can lead to sensory and motor changes in muscle, viscera, blood vessels and skin. These effects can be detected in particular areas of skin associated with the nerve roots of an inflamed branch of the pudendal nerve. This can lead to external tissue dysfunction and is known as subcutaneous panniculosis. These effects can also be detected in the presence of myofascial trigger points (sensitive focal points in the underlying muscle).

Trained therapists tackle this reaction by applying manual myofacial trigger point release procedures, connective tissue massage and special skin rolling techniques on all sensitive and painful areas.

Another suggested contributing factor in the multi-layered presentation and management of this condition targets anxiety as a stimulus for causing pelvic pain. This concept considers that in predisposed individuals, chronic stress reactions cause muscle spasm and pain. The state of chronic constriction creates pain-referring trigger points, reduced blood flow, and an inhospitable environment for the nerves, blood vessels and structures throughout the pelvic basin. This results in a cycle of pain, anxiety and tension. The Wise-Anderson Protocol (Wise & Anderson, 2008) relies, among other techniques, on the central practice of attention training in relaxing the pelvic floor, the use of RSA (respiratory sinus arrhythmia) breathing, (being aware of your breathing rates) during Trigger Point Release, and further insights in the practice of Paradoxical Relaxation.

Food and diet rarely have been considered to be a cause of pudendal neuralgia, however, there is some evidence that glucose intolerance and certain acidic foods can trigger the symptoms; these must be considered in the overall assessment plan. There is also evidence that an anti-inflammatory style diet can ease painful symptoms, such as a Mediterranean Diet (see Chapter 3).

Once again, I mention these concepts for the sake of completeness. What is evident however is the high percentage of patients with CPPS who cannot be given a contributing etiology. Mathias et al., 1996 have stated, of nine million women in the United States who had been diagnosed with CPPS, (20% of these lasting more than a year in duration), only 39% had a confirmed diagnosis, so the majority had no obvious etiology. Similarly, approximately 95% of men diagnosed with chronic prostatitis do not have an infection. (Roberts et al., 1997). However, my research, which is documented in a later chapter, and my clinical experience, would suggest that as much as 95% of patients who present with these symptoms, and have been cleared of any urological, gynaecological or gastrointestinal cause, may be associated with **lumbar-pelvic dysfunction**.

Therefore, in the following chapters, I will explain how certain patients who have a diagnosis of Pudendal Neuropathy or its subheadings, pudendal neuralgia and PNE, may be managed as a musculoskeletal condition, particularly as it relates to pelvic dysfunction.

Consequently, as an initial priority, for these pelvic pain patients, I believe an efficient differential diagnosis should concentrate on assessing the possibility of lumbar-pelvic and sacroiliac joint dysfunction. Generally, this can be accomplished simply in the clinical setting by a skilled physiotherapist or musculoskeletal health professional. The only external investigation may include a specialised MRN to determine the possibility of the presence of real entrapment, but this, from my experience probably is rare.

Ultimately, if there is no indication that pelvic dysfunction is involved, you must, of course, continue to consider other possibilities, most of which have already been mentioned.

A word here on surgery. This should only be considered after every conservative method of treatment has been exhausted. For various reasons, a certain small percentage of cases will have such rigid nerve impingement or entrapment that surgical intervention may be the only reasonable way to go.

Summary

What should be clear by now is the complex nature of CPPS. Accordingly it is no wonder that for these patients, the mean time to the diagnosis of pudendal neuropathy (pudendal neuralgia or PNE) is about four years; they have seen 10–30 Health Professionals; have suffered innumerable invasive and non-invasive procedures; have developed significant central and peripheral sensitization with the concomitant allodynia and hyperalgesia; have developed an attitude of hopelessness and have become markedly depressed to the point of committing suicide (Weiss, 2003).

It can be realised that any compromise in the nerves ability to work effi-
ciently and effectively can potentially have serious and drastic effects. These
effects are not only physical, setting up situations of chronic pain and inherently
interfering with sexual, urological and gastric functions, they can be psycholog-
ical, social and emotional, impacting significantly on self worth, identity and
relationships. Misdiagnosed, unaddressed or inadequately treated, pelvic pain
syndromes involving the pudendal nerve and other pelvic nerves can very clearly
then contribute to unsound mental health, and can prospectively spiral a patient
into reactive depression and anxiety.

In Chapter 1 I will take you through the anatomy, musculoskeletal assessment and the treatment, followed by a discussion on continued management
and prevention.

Chapter 1

Anatomy, Biomechanics and Pathology

The three main anatomical structures we need to understand, particularly in relation to pelvic pain, are the pelvic girdle, the sacroiliac joint and the pudendal nerve. However, other nerves and joints are often associated and can also contribute to the phenomenon of pelvic pain, so I will also identify and examine their roles.

The Pelvic Girdle

The pelvis is a bony ring at the base of the vertebral column, or spine. It is comprised of four bones, the *sacrum* and the *coccyx,* which are an extension of the spine, and the two *innominate* bones, (or nameless bones) which flank either side of the sacrum. The upper section of the innominate bone is called the *ilium* (ilia means flank), and it attaches to the sacrum at the sacroiliac joint (SIJ) (see Figure 1)

Stability is achieved by maintaining compression across the ring, and is dependant on deep interosseous and long dorsal ligaments posterior to the SIJ's.

The Sacroiliac Joint

The SIJ is a synovial joint and is the largest and strongest joint of the body. It provides a dynamic and mobile link between the vertebral column and the lower limb, distributing weight down the spine, through the SIJ and down the leg (see Figures 1 and 2).

The joint basically functions as a shock absorber, being lined with tough hyaline and fibrous cartilage. It is also supported by a blending of powerful lig-

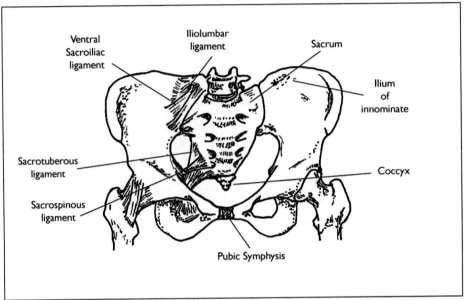

Figure 1. The Pelvis and the Sacroiliac Joint (front view)

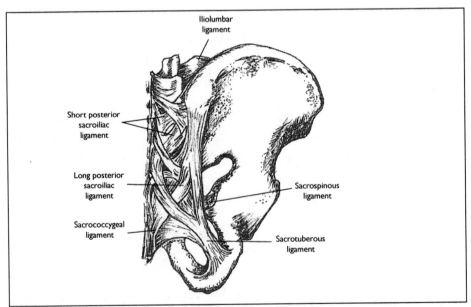

Figure 2. The Pelvis and the Sacroiliac Joint (back view)

aments and articular capsule. The articular surface is L-shaped and has developed a variety of irregular elevations and depressions. These configurations produce interlocking of the two bones which assists in creating great stability.

Of clinical interest, particularly in relation to treatment procedures using mobilising techniques, it is important to realise that the joint exhibits at least two planes of movement, often three, slightly angulated to one another.

However, while SIJ mobility has been shown to be limited, significant movement does occur (Lee, 2011). Several studies agree that the average rotation of the innominate on the sacrum in the weight-bearing position is probably less than 2.5° with about 1mm of translation. The research suggests if the joint rotates more than 6° and translates more than 2mm, pathologic changes (damage or trauma) would most probably occur.(Jacob & Kissling, 1995).

It is this mechanism which I propose may compromise the pudendal nerve. The putative reasoning suggests that if extreme physical stress causes the ilium to excessively rotate on the sacrum or the sacrum to rotate excessively on the ilium, (potentially damaging the SIJ), compression may be placed on the pudendal nerve as it moves and stretches between various pelvic anatomical structures. Most researchers and clinicians suggest that this may occur, in particular, between the sacrospinous and sacrotuberous ligaments, and in the Alcock's canal. The sacrospinous and sacrotuberous ligaments attach the sacrum to the innominates below the SIJ and are considered to be accessory ligaments. (Detachment of these ligaments by surgery apparently does not affect stability).

Compounding this situation, over and above any neural involvement, it is suggested that, as a result of excessive innominate or sacral rotation, significant soft tissue damage occurs to the SIJ ligaments. As these ligaments heal, forming fibrotic scar tissue, the joint may stiffen (in a malaligned positon) and ostensibly can result in chronic SIJ restrictions. This change in the pelvic girdle biomechanics may then exert unremitting pressure on the pudendal nerve, giving rise to serious neural symptoms, including pain and sensitisation. Assessment is aimed at revealing the particular restriction of motion where the joint is 'stuck' (see Chapter 2). The treatment is to restore that motion.

The Pudendal Nerve

The pudendal nerve gains its name from the Latin word 'pudenda', which means 'private parts,' or 'the shamefuls'. It is a mixed nerve containing somatic fibres (sensory and motor) and autonomic fibres. The autonomic fibres constitute that part of the visceral nervous system which functions automatically, affecting micturition, perspiration, sexual arousal, skin changes etc. This means the pudendal nerve has the facility to transfer messages, (hot, cold, etc) to the central nervous system. It can also transfer messages, both to control active movements, in particular to some of the pelvic floor muscles, including the bladder and bowel sphincters, as well as to control involuntary bodily functions, such as erectile ability and bladder and bowel function. In fact, the pudendal nerve is a major contributor to bladder control. Essentially, however, the pudendal nerve is mainly involved with indeed, what the ancients deemed as shameful, the sexual organs.

The pudendal nerve emerges from the sacral plexus, gaining fibres primarily from the second, third and fourth anterior sacral nerve roots (S_2 S_3 and S_4) and (autonomic) sympathetic fibres from the lower sympathetic chain. It does receive other contributions from S_1 and S_5. This is an important point, particularly considering the role of S_1 and its connections to the lumbar and sacral nerves (See Figures 3 and 4a,)

As several of the **lumbar** nerves, in particular, the inferior gluteal nerve, the tibial (medial popliteal) nerve, the common peroneal (lateral popliteal) nerve, and the perforating cutaneous nerve, and the **sacral** nerve, (posterior femoral cutaneous nerve), derive at least one connection from S_2 S_3 or S_4, the patient may also complain of pain in the lower back, groin, buttock, posterior thigh, calf or foot.

This pain may be referred either by neural convergence, by direct injury to the lumbar area, or by chronic SIJ damage impacting on L_5 S_1, thereby interfering with local emitting lumbar and sacral nerves. Given the wide range of innervation of the SIJ and its adjacent neural structures, SIJ capsular stimulation may also refer various pain patterns to the groin, buttock, thigh, calf or foot.

The pudendal nerve then follows a tortuous course outside and then through the pelvis. As such, it exits the pelvic cavity approximately 3cm below the SIJ, under the piriformis muscle and through the greater sciatic foramen, and then descends on the underside of the sacrotuberous ligament.

Early on, the inferior haemorrhoid nerve (or rectal nerve) leaves the pudendal nerve, and makes its way to supply the anal sphincter and the skin around the anus, particularly below the ischial tuberosity (connecting with the inferior cluneal nerve). The pudendal nerve then passes under the sacrospinous ligament on the inside of the ischial spine and re-enters the pelvic cavity through the lesser sciatic foramen immediately adjacent to the sacrospinous ligament.

This is the area where most researchers and clinicians speculate that the nerve has a high probable chance of being 'entrapped', between the sacrospinous and sacrotuberous ligaments.

Once the nerve has re-entered the pelvis, it travels upwards and forwards along the wall of the ischio-rectal fossa, underneath the obturator fascia. This is another area, the Alcock's Canal, within the obturator internus muscle, where it is speculated the nerve may become pinched and cause irritation.

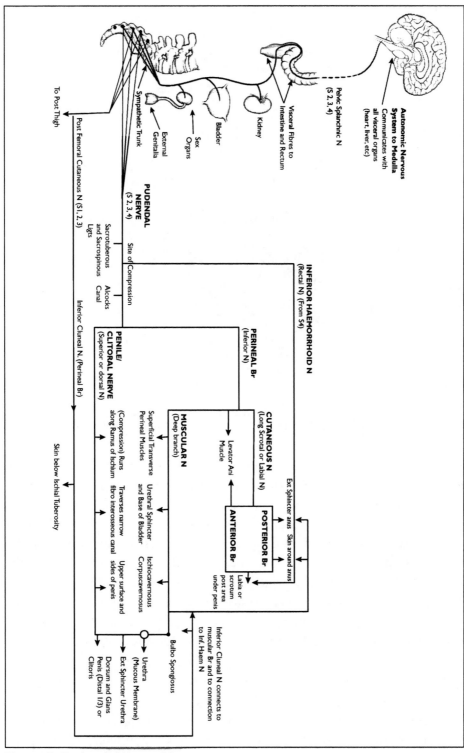

Figure 3. Pudendal Nerve Map

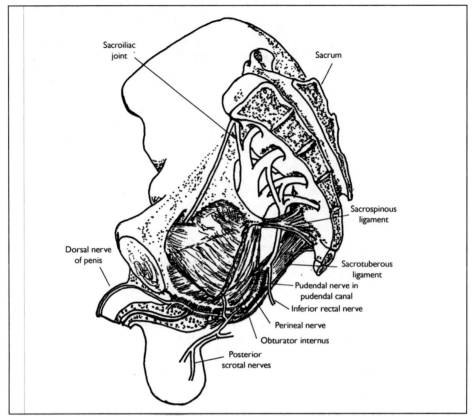

Figure 4a. The Pudendal Nerve

Neurodynamic testing can be applied here. As the obturator internus is an external rotator of the thigh, placing the leg in internal rotation may increase symptoms as the muscle and the nerve become stretched. Functionally, many patients with pudendal neuralgia cannot perform a deep squat or split squat without pain in some or all of the pudendal nerve distribution. Particularly if there is suspicion the nerve may be irritated as it moves between the sacrospinous and sacrotuberous ligaments or the Alcock's canal.

Here, the pudendal nerve divides into two terminal branches — the **inferior** (also called the **perineal** branch), and the **superior**, (also called the **penile/clitoral** branch or the **dorsal nerve)**. Researchers have noted where these two nerves leave the main trunk, after the Alcock's Canal, they do so at an angle. As mentioned earlier, they also speculate that this may increase the chances of compression and/or entrapment.

The dorsal (or superior) nerve can be endangered in this area as it runs along the ramus of the ischium (the part of the pelvis you sit on while riding a bike) towards the pubic symphysis. (It can be easily compressed here by sitting on a poor-fitting bicycle seat, resulting in penile numbness/pain). In the female, a painful allodynia response can be elicited by entering the vagina and palpating the nerve along the ischial ramus.

Further, the dorsal nerve can be endangered as it approaches the pubic symphysis in an area where it traverses a narrow fibro-interosseous canal. Researchers speculate this area may also increase the risk of compression and/or entrapment. The nerve then supplies the upper surface and sides of the penis and the dorsum and distal 1/3 of the glans, (or the clitoris). It also sends a connection, with the sympathetic nerves from the pelvic plexus (the cavernous nerve) to the muscular nerve (or deep branch) and the corpus cavernosum muscle.

Of interest, this is the same connection, with the cavernous nerve, which can lead to erectile dysfunction during prostate surgery (radical prostatectomy). It is part of the large neuro-vascular plexus which surrounds the prostate.

In the meantime, the perineal branch (or the inferior nerve), actually divides into two branches, forming the **cutaneous** branch, (or **long scrotal nerve or labial nerve),** and the **muscular** branch.

The muscular branch follows along to innervate the levator ani muscle, (which lifts the pelvic floor), most of the muscles which supply the perineum, (the area between the scrotum and the anus), the urethra (for passage of urine), and the muscles which allow erectile function (for penis and clitoris). It also sends a slip to the **inferior rectal nerve** (see Figures 3, 4a, 4b, and 4c) and one to the **inferior cluneal nerve**, (or perineal branch of the posterior femoral cutaneous nerve), which supplies the skin below the ischial tuberosity (see Figure 5).

The cutaneous branch divides into the posterior and anterior branches. The posterior branch curves below and to the back of the ischio-rectal fossa, pierces the fascia lata and runs to the skin behind the scrotum and under the area of the penis in the male and the external labia in women. Along the way it innervates the anus and the sphincter ani (the muscles which control the anus). It also communicates with the inferior haemorrhoidal nerve which, as mentioned previously, leaves the pudendal nerve very early on. This nerve supplies the skin around the anus and also the external sphincter ani (but not the actual rectum).

The anterior branch passes to the fore part of the ischio-rectal fossa and goes to the scrotum and under part of the penis (and the labia in the female). It also gives one or two filaments to the levator ani muscle.

Importantly, the pudendal nerve is also vital for erectile function in both sexes. It innervates the corpus cavernosus and corpus spongiosus muscles, the muscles which pump blood into the penis to attain an erection, and bulbo spongiosus and ischio cavernosus muscles, the muscles which maintain blood in the penis during erection, while in the female it is used for clitoral erection. It is

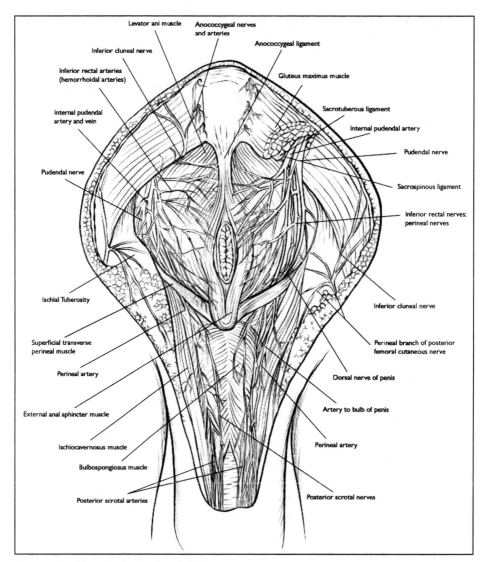

Figure 4b. The Male Pudendal Nerve

also involved with the mechanics of defaecation, ejaculation and most of the feelings of orgasm. **Orgasmic sensations** are thought to be shared between the pudendal, pelvic and vagal nerves. (Even though the actual nerve allowing orgasm comes from T11, T12, if the penis is numb [through pudendal nerve damage — sensory messages cannot get through], orgasm [and ejaculation] can not occur).

The nerve is also critical for normal bladder and bowel function, receiving both visceral and muscular fibres. Depending on the site of damage to the nerve,

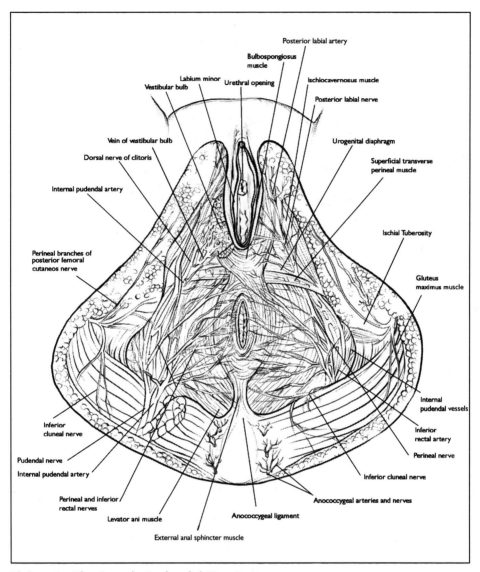

Figure 4c. The Female Pudendal Nerve

involvement here can lead to pain in either or both areas plus urinary and/or faecal incontinence and urge incontinence to either or both.

A point to remember

All of these nerves and their connections, as well as the associated ligaments have been found to have many variations. The discussion in this book therefore is a useful generality.

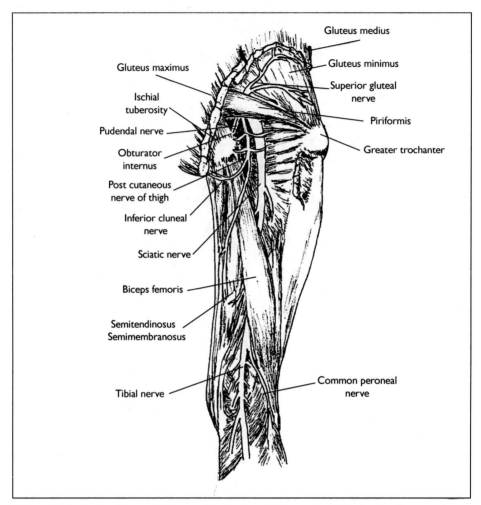

Figure 5. Inferior Cluneal Nerve (or Perineal Branch of Posterior Femoral Cutaneous Nerve)

Other Nerves, Including Thorocolumbar, Lumbar and Sacral Nerves

To reinforce the complexities involved when dealing with the pelvic neural system, several communicating lumbar nerves, (from L1 and L2) the ilio-hypogastric, ilio-inguinal and genito-femoral, also send branches to the scrotum, (or upper vulva and labia majora) (see Figure 7 page 23). They can also send branches to the upper and inner parts of the thigh. (Pain in this area is often misdiagnosed as groin, adductor muscle, hernia or pubic symphysis involvement). The genito-femoral nerve also supplies the cremaster muscle, a not-so-common area presenting as a painful symptom.

Further, the prostate and the upper part of the bladder receives its nerve supply from this same ilio-hypogastric plexus, while the base and neck of the bladder predominately receives its supply from the sacral plexus, including the pudendal nerve.

Another lumbar nerve, the obturator (from L3 and L4), can also refer pain via cutaneous branches to the outer layers of the inner thigh, the hip and medial knee. It also communicates with the deep pelvis and buttocks — the obturator externus and adductor muscles of the thigh (see Figure 7).

The largest lumbar nerve, the femoral nerve (from L3 and L4) supplies the iliacus, pectineus and the muscles on the front of the thigh, with cutaneous filaments going to the front and inner side of the thigh and to the leg and the foot. It also supplies articular branches to the front of the knee. So this nerve can also produce symptoms in the buttock, front of the thigh and knee.

Another important area to consider relates to the thoraco-lumbar region. The 10th thoracic nerve, where it leaves through the 4th sacral segments, innervate the reproductive organs, abdominal wall, low back, thighs and the pelvic floor. Also the 12th thoracic to the 4th lumbar segments can refer pain to the lower abdomen, iliopsoas, quadratus lumborum, piriformis and obturator internus muscles.

Along these lines, one explanation for some of the symptoms is that they may be caused by a dysfunction in the thorocolumbar junction as described by Maigne (Maigne, 1980; Maigne 1981). Maigne stated that referred pain from spinal nerves T_{12} and L_1 can manifest itself as low back pain which mimics pain of lumbosacral or sacroiliac origin. Referred pain from spinal nerves originating from here can also be felt in the lower abdomen, the medial aspect of the upper thigh and the groin, labia majora or scrotum. Treatment in this case includes spinal manipulation of the thorocolumbar region, and, Maigne suggests, infiltration of the painful zygapophysial joint with a corticosteroid.

To complete the review, another sub-group of patients report pain in sitting, which is relieved by standing and peculiarly, by sitting on a toilet seat. This is generally caused by pressure being applied to a branch of the posterior femoral cutaneous nerve (or posterior cutaneous nerve of the thigh). The posterior femoral cutaneous nerve itself arises from S1, S2, and S3 and provides innervation to the skin of the posterior surface of the thigh and leg, as well as to the skin of the lateral perineum, labia majora and clitoris. The particular branch, the perineal branch (or inferior cluneal nerve) swings medially below the ischial tuberosity and refers pain to the upper and medial side of the gluteal muscle and thigh and to the perineum. Thus, while sitting on a toilet seat, there will be much reduced, or no pressure, on this nerve as the pressure is applied laterally (off the sensitive area).

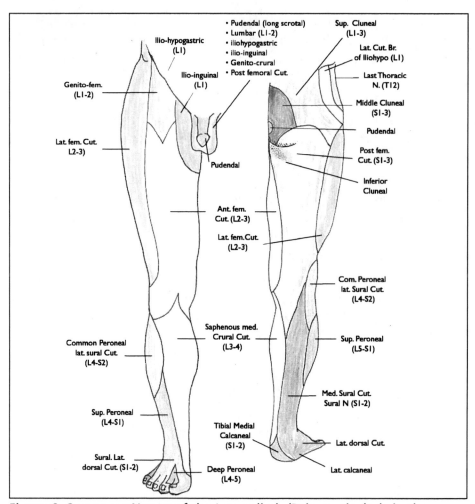

Figure 6. Cutaneous Nerves of the Lower limb (Pain particularly in the scrotal skin)

As with the pudendal nerve, Darnis, Robert and Labat (Darnis, Robert & Labat, 2008) have documented that the inferior cluneal nerve can be compressed at the level of the sacrotuberous ligament and it can also be compromised along its passage under the ischium.

The management here initially is to look for a SIJ dysfunction. This is in case the post cutaneous nerve of the thigh is compromised at its origin, S1, S2 and S3. Begin by mobilising the SIJ (as per *Treatment* in Chapter 3), then aim to desensitise the nerves by reducing pressure on them while sitting. Always sit on a "modified" type of seat, (a personalised cushion with the centre and front section removed) or simply stand if possible. If that doesn't settle the symptoms,

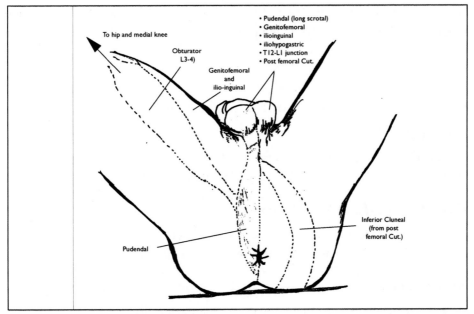

Figure 7. Innervation of the Perineum

arrange for an MRN of the inferior cluneal nerve to test for local damage (or entrapment) here.

The other nerves to consider are the superior cluneal (L1, L2, L3) which innervates the skin of the upper and lateral part of the buttocks, and the middle cluneal nerves (S1, S2, S3) which supplies the middle area of the buttocks (see Figure 6). Clinicians have noticed that these cluneal nerves can be restricted in their osteofibrous tunnels. The initial conservative treatment should be to mobilise the appropriate joints L1, L2, L3 or S1, S2 and S3. Active surgical release is a common treatment for all three cluneal nerves.

Of interest to men who suffer scrotal pain, (and this is 80% of men who I see with pudendal neuralgia), and women who have labia or vulva pain, the long scrotal nerve (labial nerve for females) is probably the main offending culprit. However, the difficulty in diagnosing the origin of scrotal pain (or labia pain) is clearly obvious. As has been detailed previously, many nerves actually communicate with the scrotum (or labia):

- Long scrotal nerve (or labial nerve) — of the pudendal nerve
- Lumbar nerves (ilio–hypogastric, ilio- inguinal and genito-crural-L1-L2)
- Thoroco–lumbar junction, T_{12}, L_1 (Maigne's Syndrome)
- Posterior-femoral cutaneous nerve (S1,S2,S3) via the inferior cluneal nerve.

Regardless, an investigation into the possibility of pelvic dysfunction, lumbar spinal involvement or Maigne's Syndrome will generally address most of these cases. (Note: The testes [and ovary], epididymis and vas deferens are innervated by thorocolumbar nerve roots T10–T11.)

Overview of nerve distribution to major anatomical areas

Penis and clitoris

Shaft and glans (tip of head of penis) and clitoris — penile or clitoral branch (superior or dorsal nerve) of the pudendal nerve.

Erectile tissue of penis and clitoris

The cavernous nerves (sympathetic system) and the muscular nerve (deep branch) of the perineal branch (inferior nerve) of the pudendal nerve.

Scrotum and labia

- The long scrotal or labial nerve of the perineal branch (inferior nerve) of the pudendal nerve.
- Lumbar nerves (ilio-hypogastric, ilio-inguinal, and genito-femoral nerves L1-2).
- Thoraco-lumbar junction, T12–L1 (Maigne's Syndrome).
- Posterior femoral cutaneous nerve (S1,2,3) via the inferior cluneal nerves.

Epididymus, testes and ovary

T10–T11.

Perineum – levator ani and superficial transverse perineal muscles.

Muscular nerve (deep branch) of perineal branch (inferior nerve) of pudendal nerve.

Lower part of abdomen

Ilio-hypogastric, ilio-inguinal and genito-femoral nerves L1-2.

Base of bladder and urethral sphincter

For urge incontinence and suprapubic pain. Muscular nerve (deep branch) of perineal branch (inferior nerve) of pudendal nerve.

Prostate and upper part of bladder

Hypogastric plexus

Anus

For faecal urgency and pain at external sphincter and skin around the anus – from the posterior branch of the cutaneous nerve (long scrotal and labial nerve) of the pudendal nerve and the inferior haemorrhoid nerve (rectal nerve).

Ischial Tuberosity

Skin below the ischial tuberosity and to perineum — from the inferior cluneal nerve (perineal branch) of the posterior femoral cutaneous nerve.

Upper and Inner parts of the thigh

The lumbar nerves (L1 and L2) — ilio-hypogastric, ilio-inguinal and genito-femoral. Also T12-L1 junction.

Chapter 2

Musculoskeletal Assessment

A s has been stated, there can be many causes of pelvic pain. It is possible a significant percentage of these can be attributed to compromise of the pudendal nerve. Revealing an accurate diagnosis may initially involve a multifaceted approach. This may include assessments and investigations by health professionals from urology, gynaecology, gastroenterology, neurology, pain management, pelvic floor physiotherapists and recently from professionals with a special interest in musculoskeletal health.

Once medical practitioners have cleared the cause as not being related to something local or systemic, or something which they can treat, the patient should be referred to a musculoskeletal therapist for further examination.

It is important to be alert to the section on musculoskeletal conditions highlighted by Prendergast and Rummer (on Page 5) which could potentially be associated with pudendal neuralgia. However, I strongly recommend, initially, the therapist should search for clues implicating lumbar-pelvic dysfunction, in particular, malalignment of either of the innominate bones on the sacrum. What we are searching for is evidence that one or both of the innominates may be significantly rotated on the sacrum, a situation which may cause compression to be placed on the pudendal nerve.

There is an admitted risk with this direct approach that the therapist may invoke 'confirmational bias' — that is, you may find what you are searching for.

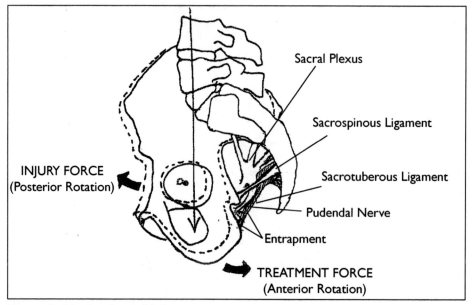

Figure 8. Mechanism of Injury

A certain percentage of the population probably have a degree of pelvic dysfunction regardless and not demonstrate pudendal neuralgia symptoms. However, the risk is justified by the research documented in Chapter 4.

Theoretically, a strong enough force on the pelvis in **any** direction could change the mechanics in relation to the path of the nerve. Realistically, the most common force which will do this is one which posteriorly rotates the innominate on the sacrum, such as in sitting or during an event which causes extreme flexion of the lower extremity (see Figure 8).

Patient History

As with all assessments the patient history can reveal important indications. Be alert for clearly relevant histories, ones that involve pelvic rotation, such as:

- An event involving fast, violent action that could rotate either of the innominates on the sacrum, such as experiencing a 'jink' in his/her back, an effect similar to that caused by stepping on a stair that's 'not there' or is lower than expected, or jumping off a train or bus. Patients often recall a sensation like a lightning electrical shock.

- Activities involving deceleration, changing direction or swivelling on one foot. Such movements which could occur at squash, tennis, soccer — (in fact, all high impact sports, including basketball, volleyball etc).

The reality here is that the patient may not immediately have associated this event with their pudendal neuralgia symptoms. Further, the patient may not have actually felt any significant back pain at the time, being generally warmed up, focussed and pumping adrenaline. During the incident, there may have been an awareness of something 'going', but only later may actual back pain be experienced, if at all; low grade, strong, protective muscle spasm of the erector spinae and hip flexor muscles often mask any significant signs of back pain and potential sacro-iliac joint involvement. In fact, the first symptom the patient may experience may be one of the symptoms or signs of pudendal neuralgia, for instance scrotal pain, which may have occurred instantly (and not that difficult to relate to the particular event), or most often, some days or weeks later; (which is more difficult to relate to pelvic involvement or a particular event). It is proposed that this is because the damaged SIJ is maintained in a malaligned position by the stiffening of fibrous tissue at the SIJ. A common presentation here is of tight iliopsoas muscles, tight piriformis muscles and tight, spasmed pelvic floor muscles. Careful questioning is needed here to match the onset of the symptoms with a possible causative event and/or back pain.

- Bending down quickly to pick up something off the floor, tying up shoe laces, bending over in the garden, cleaning, or vacuuming.

- The previous cause could be exacerbated by lifting something while bending over, such as tables, chairs, computers, cabinets, gardening pots and shovelling etc. or grandparents picking up a child, (untrained and unfit for the event).

- Sitting can bring on and/or exacerbate symptoms. This can especially affect people who sit for long periods of time, particularly if they do so without an appropriate lumbar support. IT workers and many office workers often sit for ten hours a day without adequate breaks, as do pilots, truck, taxi and courier drivers, and addicted television viewers.

- Motor vehicle accidents involving severe trauma to the pelvis, causing fractures, dislocations and rotations. Similarly, falls off bicycles (or any fall, for that matter), onto the pelvis, back, hip. A fall onto the knee can also transfer pressure to the SIJ resulting in joint damage and subsequently restrictions.

- Cyclists who spend long periods bending over low handle bars, forcing the innominates into a sustained position of extreme posterior rotation. (Note, any pudendal nerve involvement in this instance is different from that caused by sitting on an ill-fitting bicycle seat which may compress the penile branch of the pudendal nerve against the ischial ramus of the pelvis — the symptom in this case is generally numbness or pain in the penis and is initially treated by cessation of cycling or changing the seat).

- Sports involving extreme flexion of the spine — such as performing deep squats with heavy weights. This can cause the innominate to excessively posteriorly rotate on the sacrum.

- Sex. Violent, athletic and extreme actions, particularly during orgasm, causing the innominates to excessively rotate on the sacrum.

- Surgery. It is possible to inadvertently place severe rotatory stress on the SIJ during any surgery where the pelvic girdle has been sustained in an extreme or unsupported position, especially lithotomy position. (Note that surgery can also compromise the pudendal nerve from incisions, compression from retractors, suture ligature and scarring: these causes **won't** be assisted by pelvic dysfunction treatment).

- This previous situation, of course, can also occur during exhaustive sleep, or whilst under the influence of drugs or alcohol. In these cases, an individual can suffer any type and degree of neuropathy, particularly palsy to nerves of the brachial or sciatic plexuses. (During healthy sleep, nature intends an individual to roll or change position 40–50 times a night in order to take stress off muscles, tendons, ligaments, blood vessels, nerves etc.). As with the effects of anaesthetics during surgery, in these situations, it is possible to compromise the pudendal nerve as the dead weight of the body can place exceptional pressure on the sacroiliac joints.

- The pudendal nerve symptoms are often associated with and accompanied by low back pain, buttocks, thigh or leg pain. This low back pain and limb pain is generally a somatic referred pain. Somatic pain is generated from a somatic structure (joint, muscle tendon, disc). The pain is often deep and hard to localise and can move from area to area. This is unlike radicular pain which is due to irritation of a spinal nerve root or dorsal root ganglion. The most common cause of radicular pain is an acute disc prolapse, which will generally start in the buttock and can be a normal non-dermatodinal line from start to finish.

Sometimes, on questioning, the patient can recall that both the pudendal neuralgia symptoms and back symptoms started about the same time, but it is rare for them to have previously connected their possible relationships. Most times, the stress on the innominates and sacroiliac joints have been slow and subtle, (years of sitting incorrectly perhaps), that significant low back pain does not always occur.

In fact, for many situations, no matter what the cause, low grade muscular spasm may protect the back against pain. This muscle spasm — hypertonus, triggers articular-muscular reflexes which maintains the erector muscles in a sustained poor postural position. Further, sometimes the original traumatising event may have occurred so long ago (many years), the back (SIJ) injury will have healed and the resultant fibrous tissue will have stiffened, also helping to maintain the joint in a restricted position. This can occur to the extent where the patient does not necessarily, at this stage, complain of back pain. He may not even complain of stiffness, but that is what your further examination and questioning will search for — SIJ back pain and/or stiffness.

Physical Assessment

Researchers have consistently reported that the clinical diagnosis of symptomatic SIJ remains problematic. Although they concede that sacroiliac joint pain is common in patients with low back pain, they believe it can only be definitively diagnosed using diagnostic local anaesthetic blocks. However, there is agreement that combined provocative clinical tests may be useful.

One of the problems appears to be that most provocative clinical tests evaluate either function or pain, which of course, may not equate to each other, and certainly may not adequately equate to SIJ damage consistent to trigger a varied plethora of pudendal neuralgia symptoms.

My experience is that most patients who present with a diagnosis of pudendal neuralgia, (which has not been attributed to an obvious urological, gynaecological, gastroenterological or neurological cause), may, on examination, be found to have either SIJ pain and/or dysfunction, or both. However, vexingly, some patients, particularly patients with chronic pudendal neuralgia symptoms, may be found to have no SIJ pain, and only minimal dysfunction, often so minimal that they have not been aware of it.

Sometimes, testing may reveal tight iliopsoas muscles, piriformis tension and tight, painful pelvic floor muscles. Trigger point massage and other relaxation techniques can often relieve these symptoms, but rarely relieve the pudendal neuralgia symptoms. (In fact, because the pelvic floor muscles are supplied by the pudendal nerve, trigger point massage often exacerbates symptoms). Therefore, I consider that in some cases, ones where provocative clinical tests do not reveal significant pain and/or dysfunction, another criterion must be introduced.

What I propose now arises from a purely clinical observation. I submit that what we really have to look for here is SIJ **stiffness** — often so little stiffness that it may not show up effectively with any pain, functional or provocational tests.

As previously proposed, I consider for the SIJ to be involved in the cause of pudendal neuralgia, one (or both) of the innominates has to be appreciably restricted in its movement on the sacrum. In this regard, the **history** may already have alerted us and revealed perhaps a pertinent specific event, or poor seating posture, which may be associated with this possibility.

Therefore, with all this in mind, the real key, I believe, to implicate SIJ involvement is to search for joint stiffness. This is done by using palpation to thoroughly explore the joint. It is not dissimilar to classic 'Spring Tests' used for Motion Grading to test actual mobility in the joint.

If the injury is significant, such as related to a specific, notable event, and recent (within six weeks), palpation over the SIJ will generally be reactive, painful and stiff. However, if the examination is carried out many months, or even years, after the causative event, the body (and brain) may have adapted to this new situation and clinically, there may be no notable dysfunction or pain. The only finding may be localised joint stiffness, which may only be revealed on sensitive and creative palpation. Generally, this will be a posterior to anterior glide force of about 10 pounds (about 4.7 kilograms) to take up the slack, then additional 10 pounds to 'spring' or get to the 'end feel' (Hesch, 2011).

I have found it useful to refer to Maitlands classic mobilisation grading (Maitland, 2005). I note degrees of pain and stiffness as:

>   Grade I — small amplitude
>
>   Grade II — larger amplitude
>
>   For stiffness only — (no irritability)
>
>   Grade III — large amplitude
>
>   Grade IV — small end of range of movement amplitude

This, of course, is useful for recording the status of the joint at the initial assessment, and also to acknowledge the effectiveness of ongoing treatment.

A small warning here: some patients with chronic pelvic pain symptoms who have been on various medications for pain relief (and for other co-morbidities, high cholesterol etc) can present with a swollen, often bloated abdomen. Initially be aware that aggressive palpation over the SIJ may inflame symptoms.

To appreciate the rationale for, and the validity of this test, a deeper understanding of the process of the pathology of healing and regeneration, as discussed briefly in Chapter 1, is necessary. Simply, in the early inflammatory and fibroblastic phases of healing, usually the first few weeks, fibroblasts replace the damaged ligaments with fibrous tissue and aggregate into collagen fibres, an activity which may eventually take from six to ten weeks.

As the healing process moves into the final stage — the maturation phase — remodelling of the wound develops the collagen fibres into a stronger weave, a process which may require six to twelve months. This fibrous tissue (scar tissue) however, is less extensible, the joint becomes stiff, potentially malaligning the innominate on the sacrum. (Of importance, experience and documentation has shown that it is possible to minimise the negative effects of this process. Early intervention, such as appropriate exercise and mobilisation, can influence and control fibrosis and limit dysfunction by remodelling and 'unwinding' the scar tissue fibres).

When testing for stiffness, it is important to remember that motion of the pelvic girdle is triplanar. That is, movement can occur in all three body planes — flexion/extension, side flexion and axial rotations, producing potential for six degrees of freedom. However, as noted earlier, the SIJ is only capable of limited rotational and translational movement in one plane. Therefore, it is not difficult to imagine how, when **great** stress is applied from any of the above mentioned planes, theoretically, any part or combination of parts of any of the ligaments which stabilise the SIJ could be injured.

Further, the SIJ is 'L' shaped, much like a boomerang with one arm shorter than the other. Therefore, it is important to thoroughly search and palpate in any and every direction you can creatively manage. Keeping in mind, as mentioned earlier, the joint can exhibit two, or even three, planes of movement.

When stiffness is found, this situation is often referred to as the joint being 'out', 'malaligned', 'fixated', or 'excessively compressed'.

The other area which is useful to test is the coccyx. While a fall on the coccyx can potentially rotate the sacrum on the innominate, it can also strain or dislocate the coccyx on the sacrum, damaging the connecting ligaments. As fibres from both the sacrotuberous and sacrospinous ligaments attach to the coccyx, and the pudendal nerve moves between the sacrotuberous and sacrospinous ligaments, it is possible to create significant compression on the pudendal nerve.

It is therefore important to test the coccyx by palpation for pain and/or stiffness.

Chapter 3

Treatment

T he musculoskeletal treatment to manage symptoms of pudendal neu-ropathy, particularly in relation to the SIJ, is approached in four phases:

1. The primary aim of treatment is to release the restrictions maintaining the innominate on the sacrum in an incorrect position. This is achieved initially by manual mobilising and manipulative techniques, then by exercises.

2. It is imperative to teach the patient how to maintain the correct and optimal lumbar posture, particularly whilst sitting.

3. There may be a need to understand and manage chronic pain cycles and neural hypersensitivity.

4. A prevention program should be instituted by maintaining an appropriate exercise program and being constantly aware of the importance of correct posture.

Release the restrictions maintaining the innominate in an incorrect position on the sacrum

There are many possible presentations of SIJ dysfunction, (involving abnormal rotation of the innominate on the sacrum), that may cause Pudendal Neuropathy, pudendal neuralgia or pudendal nerve entrapment and its associated symptoms. The immediate aim of treatment in all cases is to realign the innominate on the sacrum.

The most common presentation is one where the innominate is rotated posteriorly on the sacrum (See Figure 8, page 28). The aim of treatment, in this case, is to 'release' the innominate by rotating it anteriorly. This is achieved in three stages; (1) heating the tissues, (2) mobilising the SIJ manually and (3) exercises.

Heat

Heat is applied to the SIJ and to the tissues in the surrounding areas. The main effects of heat in this instance, are:

1. To relieve pain in the joint and the surrounding tissues. It is found that a mild degree of heating is effective in relieving pain, presumably as a result of a sedative effect on the sensory nerves.

2. To relieve protective muscle spasm. By virtue of relieving pain, associated muscle spasm and tension are also relieved.

3. To increase extensibility of the collagen fibres of the scar tissue. When considering the reaction of heat on soft tissue, it has been shown that temperature has a significant influence on the mechanical behaviour of connective tissue under tensile stress. As tissue temperature rises, stiffness decreases and extensibility increases. Both applied heat and exercise can produce a temperature rise.

4. To enhance easier mobilising/stretching routines and to facilitate muscle contractility.

In the therapist's rooms, shortwave and microwave diathermy penetrate deeply and produce as much as five to six degrees increase in temperature to a depth of 5 centimetres. At home, heat packs, infrared lamp, hot water bag, warm showers and baths are all effective.

Mobilisation — manual mobilising and manipulative techniques.

Basically, the term mobilisation refers to a stretching process designed to increase the range of movement of a stiff joint. It is a collective term incorporating two techniques, *mobilisation* and *manipulation*. *Mobilisation* can be applied as passive small or large oscillatory movements, two or three a second, anywhere in a range of movement and it can also be applied as a sustained stretch at the limit of the range. *Manipulation* describes a sudden movement or thrust, of small amplitude and high speed, at the end of the range.

Mobilisation can be achieved by the therapist manually applying 'passive movement' techniques to the joint, (Figure 9) or by the patient actively performing specific exercises.

For the SIJ the aim of mobilisation is to restore structures within the joint to their normal position so as to recover a full-range painless movement.

Initially, once the therapist has identified specific stiff structures within the SIJ, small amplitude passive movement techniques are used to mobilise the SIJ. This will take some creativity as the therapist must search for stiff sections in all ligamentous, fibrotic and fascial structures and tissues which make up the SIJ. This will include any spin, roll or slide features which are normal for the joint. This will also mean searching for, and mobilising, any adaptive stiffening of any other related joint structures.

As the joint shows signs that this technique is gradually increasing mobility, the therapist may then introduce a slow, stronger, stretching technique holding in a sustained position for about 10–15 seconds building up to at least a minute, even two minutes. Do not stint on time here, or pressure. We are trying to change the quality of scar tissue restrictions by utilising principles of **visco-elastic creep** (Hesch, 2011). Creep is an important concept when treating isolated SIJ mobility. It is known that treatment forces held steady against a motion barrier (adhesions, spasm) for several minutes will induce tissue relaxation resulting in an increase in joint mobility and soft tissue extensibility. The tissue is taken beyond the elastic limit inducing plastic (more

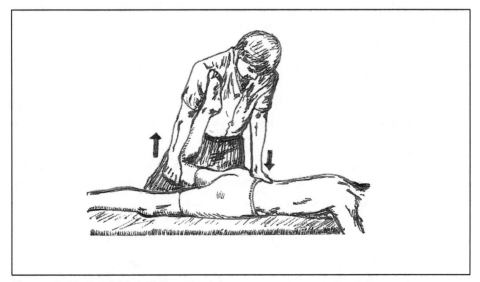

Figure 9. Manual Mobilising Stretch

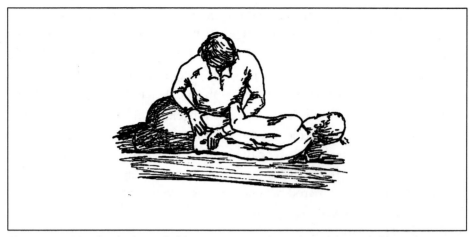

Figure 10. Manipulation of the SIJ — Posterior Distraction of the Left SIJ

lasting) deformation. Clinically, the scarring is fundamentally altered. A special technique for this presentation is to stretch the SIJ by rotating the innominate anteriorly (see also Figure 9).

With the patient lying prone close to the edge of the table, the therapist supports the anterior aspect of the distal thigh with one hand and lifts the hip into extension, while the posterior superior iliac spine of the innominate is palpated with the heel of the other hand. The limit of anterior rotation of the innominate is reached by passively extending the hip with one hand and applying an anterior rotation force to the innominate with the other hand. The pressure is held for 15 seconds, building up to a minute or more on full stretch.

This effect can be enhanced by applying a manipulative technique to the SIJ (see Figure 10).

With the patient in right side lying, lower leg extended and upper hip and knee flexed, the thoraco-lumbar spine is fully rotated to the left. Find the stiffest level of resistance. The therapist stabilises the sacrum with one hand while the other hand applies a high velocity, low amplitude thrust through the left innominate.

Although researchers are not sure of the exact mechanism underlying the effects of this technique, it is considered to be effective to restore joint mobility, for whatever reason (Lee, 2011).

Exercises

Exercises are important, not just to maintain the joint range of movement or to regain the flexibility, strength and endurance components of the muscles which control the joint, but to restimulate joint and muscle mechano-receptors. The following exercises should be performed at least once a day. As scarring contracts/stiffens with inactivity, the injured areas will generally be at their stiffest first thing in the morning. This is the recommended time to run through these.

(a) **Hip Rolls**. Patient lying supine, legs hip width apart, lift the buttocks to a long diagonal line between the shoulders, hips and knees. Roll or glide the pelvis to one side, back to the middle, then the other. Return to the middle and lower buttocks to the floor. 10 repetitions. (See Figure 11)

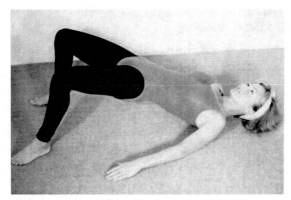

Figure 11. Hip Rolls

(b) **Low Back Stretch.** Patient lying supine, use two hands to draw one thigh and knee to the chin, keeping the other leg flat and extended. Hold this thigh on strong overpressure for 5 seconds and release. Repeat 5 repetitions each leg. (See Figure 12)

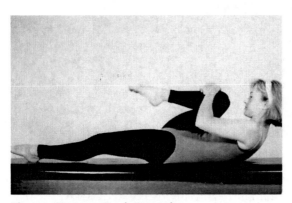

Figure 12. Low Back Stretch

(c) **Full Spine Strengthening.** Patient kneeling on all fours, hands underneath shoulders, knees under hips, Flex and stretch one knee towards the chin, then extend head and leg. Repeat 10 times each leg. (See Figure 13)

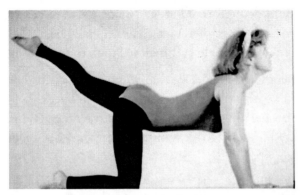

Figure 13. Full Spine Strengthening

(d) **SIJ Stretch.** Patient kneeling on a chair with elbows placed on strong table. One leg (knee) is positioned over the edge of the chair and hooked over the other leg for support. The forementioned leg is stretched fully below the edge of the chair and held in position here for 5 seconds, then lifted fully higher than the edge of the chair and held here for five seconds. This is repeated each side 10 times. (See Figure 14)

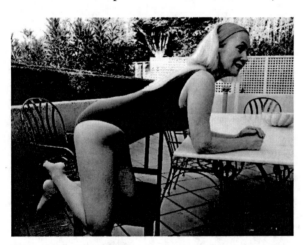

Figure 14. SIJ Stretch

(e) **Abdominal (core) Exercises.** Patient in supine, knees flexed, feet flat on floor, hands behind head and supporting neck. Draw the navel to the floor to flatten abdominals, and then raise head and shoulders, (as in 'crunches'). Repeat 6 times. Then, as the patient sits up, rotate the trunk towards one knee, repeat 6 times, then repeat to the other knee 6 times. (See Figure 15 a & b)

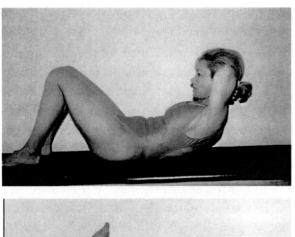

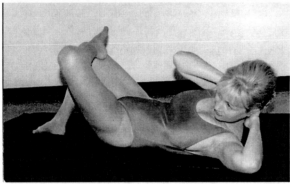

Figure 15. a & b. Abdominal (core) Exercises

Maintaining the Correct Lumbar Posture

Incorrect posture, particularly in sitting, is probably the major underlying cause of the endemic incidence of spinal pain in Western society. It can certainly be the cause of certain presentations of Pudendal Neuropathy. By the time we reach our late thirties, the physical consequences of a lifetime of sedentary occupations, particularly IT related, hobbies, and television habits become obvious.

There's a curve to our posture that wasn't there before. The head begins to slump forward, changing the entire balance of the body. The head weighs 5 kilograms. This is the amount of stress placed on the neck when the head is perched squarely on a person with good posture while standing erect. (see Figure 16). When the head slumps forward 2cms, the stress on the neck doubles — when it slumps forward 4cms, it quadruples — effectively increasing the stress on the neck to 20 kilograms.

Our shoulders, become more rounded. Our chest, or breasts (which can weigh 2–3 kilograms each), sag, our belly protrudes, and to compensate for the weight of the head being pushed forward, the body deepens the curve in the lumbar spine, increasing stress on it (see Figure 16).

Poor sitting posture reverses the normal curves of the spine in the regions of the neck and lower back. This situation produces a prolonged stretch to the ligaments of the spine. It is like stretching an elastic band to its extreme until it frays, then breaks. This prolonged stretch produces micro-stress trauma to all the spinal structures, and they respond by scarring and shortening (see Figure 17). It is this situation which can stress and damage the sacroiliac joints as the pelvis rotates, forcing the innominates to posteriorly rotate on the sacrum.

Poor posture is becoming increasingly evident in our children and adolescents, particularly in the slouching position they adopt in standing and sitting. Postural defects worsen with age as the effects of sedentary life (lack of exercise, poor diet, overweight, obesity and stress), take their toll.

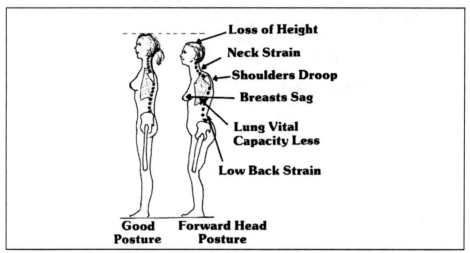

Figure 16. The Importance of Good Posture

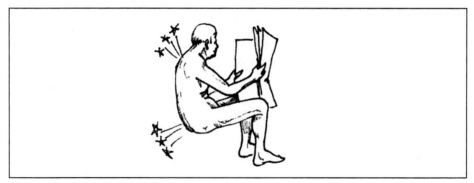

Figure 17. Poor Seating Posture

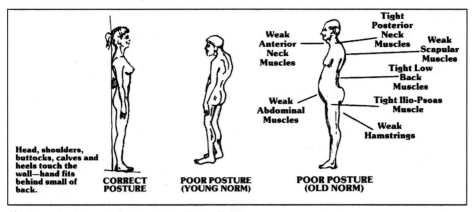

Figure 18. Correct Posture to Poor Posture

Note the change from correct posture in Figure 18, to poor posture (as in Young Norm) to 40-year-old Norm. This exaggerated diagram is becoming the caricature of 21st Century Person, the 'Norm' of everyday life.

Correct Posture Management

The postural strategies to manage and prevent symptoms of Pudendal Neuropathy and pudendal neuralgia are the same as those for managing back pain. It is critical that you become aware of your posture. If you examine your spinal column from the side, you will notice it has evolved to form an efficient spring shape. If this shape is altered extremely, the spine may be injured. **Try and maintain this natural curve in its optimal position during all changes of posture.**

Retrain the Brain

After some years of poor postural practices, the brain actually becomes programmed to believe it is normal for the head to be jutting forward, the shoulders to be rounded and the low back and pelvis to be excessively rotated. The first step in regaining correct posture is to retrain the brain to be aware of where it should be.

All you need to do is STAND TALL. Lift your head and push it to the ceiling (as demonstrated by the woman in Figure 18). It's something you can do anytime. Have deliberate posture checks regularly — at least twice daily. Think about standing tall. Imagine, if you like, you are balancing a book or weight on the top of your head. Try and keep it high. One of the most effective times to do this is on arising in the morning, when joints, muscles and tendons will generally be at their stiffest. As well, write "P" (for posture) on your desk or watch, or schedule for a regular reminder to be flagged on your computer.

Sitting Posture

When sitting, make sure all parts of your low back and neck are supported. You may have to place a cushion behind your low back to keep the curve in its natural and optimal shape (see Figure 19). Be sure not to rotate the pelvis excessively in either direction. If the chair is low, and your knees are higher than your buttocks, you may also need to place a cushion under your buttocks. You don't have to use a straight back chair — just a comfortable, supportive one. Do this when driving, watching TV, sitting at work or at home at the dinner table. Further, you are advised to change your posture every 30 minutes, even if you have no pain — stand up and walk around regularly. Keep reminding the brain of correct postural patterns.

Prolonged neck bending can lead to pain and headaches from excess strain and eventually, may lead to early degeneration of the spine. Do not have your head leaning forward for long periods, especially when at the computer (especially a laptop), reading or knitting. Desk and work-bench heights must also be arranged to prevent excessive forward tilt of the neck. In general, if your head bends further than 30 degrees forward, you have a greater risk of developing neck pain. Remember the advice at the beginning of this section; it is worth repeating — your head weighs about 5kg (12lb). If your head leans forward 2cms, the stress on your neck virtually doubles in weight (now 10kg); if you lean over 4cms, it quadruples (now 20kg or 48lbs). This pressure can eventually be thrust onto your lower back, potentially causing or exacerbating the pudendal nerve symptoms (see Figure 20).

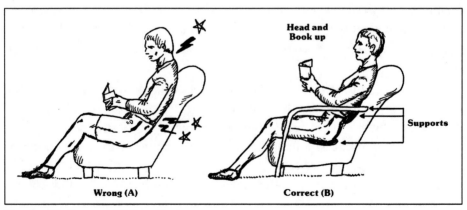

Figure 19. Correct Sitting Posture

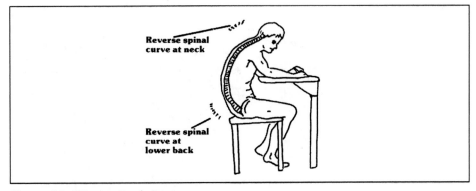

Figure 20. Wrong Desk Posture

When sitting at your computer work station, your hips should be as far back in your chair as possible. Adjust the backrest so it fits snugly in the small of your back or use a lumbar roll. Your keyboard should be relatively close to your body and directly in front of you so your forearms rest on the desk. Your seated elbow height should be approximately the same height as the desk. Your neck should be in a neutral position, so place the keyboard and screen directly in front. The optimum position for the computer screen is 15 to 50 degrees below the horizontal line of sight-not at eye level (University of Queensland, 2009). Your thighs should be parallel to the floor and your knees and ankles should be about 90 degrees (see Figure 21).

Your feet should be well supported on the ground. Laptops are difficult to use and maintain correct posture for sustained periods of comfortable use — limit laptops, or connect to an external screen.

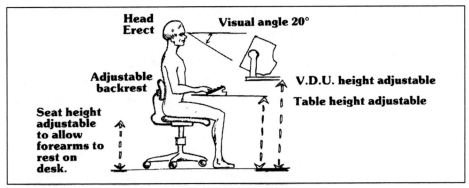

Figure 21. Correct Computer Workstation Posture

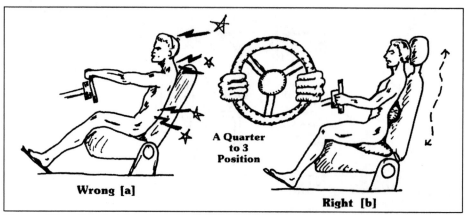

Figure 22. a & b Driving Posture

Driving

When driving, there are four main points to follow to prevent neck and back pain.

1. The hip and knees should be parallel to the ground. Often modern low cars are designed with the front of the seat higher than the back (as in Figure 22). You may need to add a cushion under your rear for support (see Figure 22b).

2. Arrange the car seat close to the steering wheel, with the back rest adjusted as near as possible to the upright position.

3. If the seat is fitted with an adjustable lumbar support, this should be positioned to comfortably support the inwards curve of the lower back. If there is not adequate lumbar support, use a small pillow, towel or commercial lumbar support (see Figure 22b). This is critical for managing PN.

4. The steering wheel should be gripped as low down as possible (the recommended safety position is a quarter to three — ten to two is ok). If the hands are held too high on the wheel, the weight of the arms will quickly overload the neck.

When driving long distances, get out of the car regularly — at least every hour — and walk around for a minimum of 5 minutes. Stretch the neck and back muscles deliberately. Generally loosen up body structures and increase circulation.

Toilet

When "pushing" on the toilet, keep your head up, lean forward a little, take care not to slump and try and maintain the normal lumbar curve. Place your hands onto your knees. Your knees should be slightly higher than your hips. A low footstool can be useful. Relax the lower abdomen first, then further bulge out your abdomen. If you draw the abdomen inwards to increase the intra abdominal pressure to defecate, the pelvic floor muscles automatically draw upwards. As the pudendal nerve supplies the pelvic floor muscles this can trigger pain. So it is important to relax both the pelvic floor muscles and the abdominal muscles. Sometimes it is helpful to massage the abdomen, applying strong pressure following the intestines to the bowel see Figure 23).

Standing

Prolonged standing in one position places great pressure on the lumbar spine. Shifting the weight from one foot to the other relieves this strain. At the hotel bar, keep a foot on the rail or a rung of the bar stool. Similarly, use a footrest whilst ironing (see Figure 24).

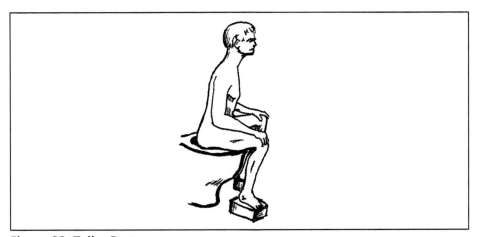

Figure 23. Toilet Posture

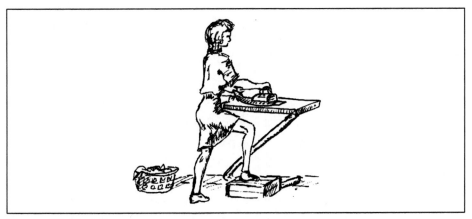

Figure 24. Standing

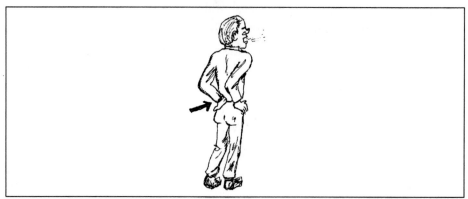

Figure 25. Sneezing, Coughing

Sneezing and Coughing

Sneeze or cough upwards, (taking care not to cough on anyone), rather than bending forwards and risk placing increased intra-abdominal and intra-pelvic pressure on the SIJ's. Arch your spine backwards and, placing your hands in the small of your back, push in to equalise the pressure as you cough and sneeze (see Figure 25).

Heavy Loads

Heavy loads should be balanced on both shoulders. If the package cannot be divided, it should be switched from side to side to relieve the lopsided pressure, for example attaché cases or babies, shopping bags etc. School children should wear proper fitting school bags or back packs if possible.

Morning Stiffness

Be careful bending over the sink for a wash first thing in the morning. The back may be stiff from sleeping — scar tissue has a tendency to contract, deform and stiffen with immobility. Maintain the low back hollow and bend the knees. (see Figure 26).

High Heel Shoes

Be wary of high-heeled shoes, as they tend to throw the spine forward by tilting the pelvis. The price of fashion does not always outweigh the price of stress to the SIJ or a flare-up of pelvic pain.

Gardening

When gardening and digging, take the strain with your legs and not your back. Use a longer handled spade or shovel to prevent bending the back. Do not bend

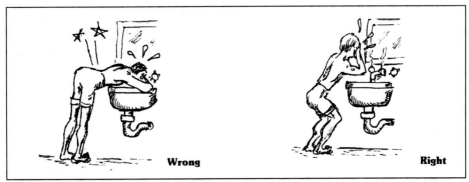

Figure 26. Morning Stiffness

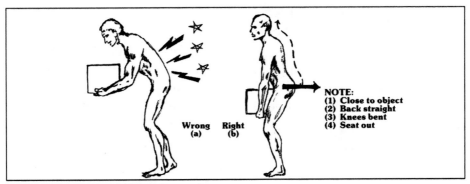

Figure 27. Correct Lifting Procedure

over while weeding. Use your whole body and kneel close to the weeds, loosening the soil first.

Lifting

When lifting, bend the knees and take the weight through the thigh muscles – they are stronger than the back. The back is not a crane. Get as close as possible to the object you are lifting, brace your abdominal muscles strongly, keep the back "straight", (as in Figure 27) and lift steadily.

Managing Chronic Pain Cycles and Neural Hypersensitivity

When managing CPPS,(Chronic pelvic pain syndrome) it is important to understand that chronic or persistent pain can develop into a disease by itself. In fact, CPPS is complex, involving multiple systems. It is about a dynamic network that includes the central nervous system (CNS), peripheral nervous system (PNS) and the end-organ. Therefore, a multidisciplinary approach may be required. A diagnosis is often reached by exclusion. We know there are many factors that can potentially interfere with normal pain modulation.

In the normal situation, animals (human beings) have developed pain as a warning, an alert concerning a stressful or threatening situation. It is a basic survival mechanism in response to a perception of threat. The process is known as nociception, and it has probably saved you countless of times. Touch a hot iron, nociceptive receptors funnel messages to your brain which responds by automatically moving away from it — fast. If we sprain an ankle, the message to the brain will be perceived as a threat and the brain will respond by protecting itself — go into a cave, do not aggravate the injury and let it heal.

In this same instant pain, (and fear of pain), will also trigger the fight/flight reflex. By secreting certain hormones, within a few seconds, the body will mobilise all systems to either punch a perpetrator, (or move the iron), or run — fast — from the stressful situation. (In fact, with the iron, nature has developed a short circuit. Instead of having to wait for the message to travel to the spine, then be transferred on to the brain, [where the brain can interpret the message then either consciously consider the threat or spontaneously react], an automatic reflex — a short circuit working locally in the spine, directs us to act — quickly. Then the hormones kick in to allow us to challenge, or not, what was threatening us).

This is pain working naturally and appropriately. Once the threatening situation has been removed, the adrenaline settles down and the painful proactive reflex cycle diminishes.

However, in the case of CPPS, there is generally an ongoing input from a persistent focus; the obstruction or stimulant causing the pain doesn't go away. If the offending structure, such as (in our alleged case) an extremely rotated pelvis, (which presumably then exerts pressure on the pudendal nerve), isn't diagnosed and therefore not adequately treated, a chronic pain cycle may develop.

This is when pain does not react appropriately. It becomes a mind/body disorder, a behavioural state with multidisciplinary connections. As stated earlier chronic pain is complex. It does not necessarily correlate with the degree of injury or disease; it is completely real and it's indistinguishable from the original pain when the nerve was originally assaulted. Psychosocial considerations can also be introduced influencing the degree of perception, including sexuality, cultural expectations, privacy and religious issues. The pain is now produced by an overly sensitised neural system which can have the effect of 'amplifying' or 'turning up' the pain.

It is important to recognise that chronic pain is not just acute pain with a longer duration. Chronic stress and pain cycles lower pain thresholds by depleting dopamine and elevating adrenaline, which in time, tightens already constricted and protective overloaded muscles. Adopting poor posture patterns, (particularly while sitting), inability to relax muscles, life stresses and lifestyle factors, sleep deficiency, hormonal shifts, depression, anxiety and dietary factors can also then disrupt normal pain modulation.

In fact, long term pain has been shown to change the plasticity of the brain. It has long been clinically observed that once the nerve structure is altered because of irritation — of any sort — the pain may persist even after the aggravating stimulus has been removed.

There is a favourite analogy for this effect. A match may start a kindling fire in the woods which may progress eventually to become a roaring forest fire. Putting out the match too late (the cause) will not stop the forest fire raging. The forest fire will develop a life of its own and need to be controlled independently.

The same applies to the nervous system. The over stimulated nerve, therefore, and its immediate neural system, is then said to become hypersensitive — a forest fire. This is called central sensitisation and plays a major role in maintaining on-going chronic pain. Any small aggravation to this over-sensitive nerve can now trigger off the pain cycle, often with "over-kill", and because of convergence between closely related nerves, often to many and varied regions.

It is not always possible to identify a particular nerve — in fact, small, unmyelenated nerve fibres are frequently responsible for this phenomenon, where functional (and measureable) changes may occur in the brain.

When a nerve is pathologically compressed or entrapped, the nerve and its branches are subject to increased friction and stretch because they are unable to slide and glide normally in their sheaths. The smallest tension placed on any part of this now sensitive nerve will be dissipated in all directions, triggering and increasing the pain cycle.

Chronic pain can sensitize (or confuse) the natural protective mechanisms of the brain, causing a chronically hyper-aroused system. This will quickly have an impact on the patients mental health causing them to lose concentration and focus. They will feel emotional and react automatically to situations, which can lead to catastrophizing (imagining the worst possible outcomes), anxiety and depression, sleep disorders and affect their sexual health and relationships.

In the case of pelvic dysfunction patients presenting with pelvic pain symptoms, the level of pain a patient experiences may then be the sum total of the joint injury, muscle spasm and associated regional myofascial trigger points, connective tissue adhesions and restrictions, neural compression, deficient pain modulators and stress, complicated by a vicious pain cycle. Management of this situation relies on determining what is the core problem driving the entire complex — treating that, then tackling any residual and persistent pain cycle.

In the context of this book, it is advised, and has already been stated, it is important to initially assess the lumbar-pelvic region, in particular the SIJ, as being the probable source of the core problem — the match that triggers, and continues to trigger, the forest fire.

If pelvic dysfunction, or SIJ rotation, is found to be the correct underlying diagnosis, and if this is then treated, it is not uncommon to find that extreme nerve sensitivity and its complications may soon markedly decrease or completely resolve, without further interventions. However, in some cases, even after treating the cause (the match) the resultant forest fire may still have a life of its own and need to be addressed — the chronic or persistent pain.

What is distressing is that with some patients, the majority of interventions such as blocks, stimulators and drugs, may eventually stop working. The neuroplasticity of the brain has been changed to view this 'forest-fire' state as a protective armament; it sees it as 'good'.

This can be changed! A few words must be said about the emerging and interesting field of study concerning neuroplasticity. Neuroplasticity is loosely defined as the brains ability to continually adapt to new information and experiences by changing its structure, function or chemistry. For example, such changes as a loss of white matter have been shown to occur in patients as a response to chronic pain. Now, research shows that relief of pain can reverse structural and functional changes and restore normal brain function.

Chronic Pain Management

For all cases of Chronic Pain Cycles and Neural Hypersensitivity, there are a number of practical ways to decrease nerve sensitisation, that is, to down–regulate an over-sensitive nervous system.

- Education — understanding the situation, an explanation of pain mechanisms, particularly the pitfalls of the recovery process in persistent pain. The patient must have ideas for taking control of recovery. Using educational tools in the clinic to accurately explain pain reduces the threat of pain. This decreases the need for the body to over-engage other coping systems by bringing in the sympathetic, immune, endocrine and motor systems.

  Knowledge is power here. The patient will gain confidence from understanding what pain is; to learn to accept that sometimes it can't be easily 'cured', and they must learn to manage it. This knowledge helps to reduce the perception of pain. They must learn to take responsibility for the pain and control how it is managed. (David Butler and Lorimer Moseley's book *Explain Pain* is an excellent resource.)

In this regard, it is also important to understand that pain can lead to depression – 'the blues'. This must be addressed as a depressed mood effectively shoots more messages to the brain which is interpreted as more pain, setting off a vicious cycle. Education (and medication) as well as controlled exercise helps to break this pain cycle, so we should focus on mood as well as pain.

- Obviously, treat the basic cause of the nerve being continually stimulated — (the match) In this case, it will be to re-align the pelvis on the sacrum (described earlier).

- Body map retraining and neuroplasticity. Research suggests that when pain positively responds to treatment, some neuroplastic brain changes regress to normal: **the changes can be reversible**! Body maps (or patterns) are the reference point for movement and sensation and constantly change with experience. The ability to undergo change is a property of plasticity of the nervous system. This can be trained as can any function, knee exercises, throwing skills etc. The idea is to address the neuromatrix by changing awareness of body parts and re-organising the sensorimotor cortex. By gradually re-engaging in normal activity, thereby getting more normal input into the brain, it is possible to begin to desensitise the hypersensitive pathways and normalise them. The following procedures can be helpful.

- Keeping active — keeping active generally will promote recovery by:
  - Avoiding disuse effects of excessive rest
  - Avoiding muscle wastage because of pain (pain actually produces atrophy faster than inactivity)
  - Regaining function and therefore independence
  - Producing natural pain-relieving chemicals-endorphins
  - Stimulate production of serotonin (the feel good hormone)
  - Retraining the nervous system
    The following routines can be helpful.
  - Gentle, rhythmic manual mobilising techniques have been found to ease pain
  - Rhythmical and gentle exercise
  - Yoga
  - Feldenkrais. Feldenkrais has developed therapeutic exercises using sensation-based movement. These can be an effective basis for gentle introductory sensory-awareness routines.

- Cardiovascular Exercise. There is well-documented evidence that aerobic exercise raises endorphin levels which has the effect of decreasing pain. It also lowers a person's stress response which assists in anxiety relief.

- Resistance Exercise. Weight training, Pilates, swimming.

- Heat, ice application

- Cognitive Behavioural therapy — challenging maladaptive cognitive structures and processes. Such techniques as distraction activities, relaxation therapy and increased engagement with pleasurable activities.

- Meditation — can help with decreasing anxiety

- Mindfulness training — learning awareness of thoughts, emotions and sensations. How we think and feel has a profound effect on all aspects of our physiology. When we are frustrated, angry, stressed, fearful, worried or depressed, everything — including pain — can seem worse.

- Positive thinking, affirmations. Patients may be able to learn to control and change their thoughts. Conversely, as thoughts are nerve impulses, negative thinking alone may drive persistent pain states.

- Guided imagery — engages the power of the mind to reduce anxiety, depression and stress.

- Hypnosis

- Relaxation training — many different techniques for this, including the Wise-Anderson Protocol, (mentioned in the Introduction).

- Good Nutrition — Diet. What you eat has a direct and immediate effect on your hormone levels, mood, pain tolerance and energy levels. The Mediterranean Diet can be effective in this regard. Besides health benefits related to managing cardiovascular disease and cancers, this diet has been considered to produce a generalised anti-inflammatory effect.

  - Emphasize fruits, dark green leafy vegetables, whole grains, legumes, nuts, seeds.

  - Eat a **rainbow** of fruits and vegetables — orange, green, yellow, red, purple, white.

  - Choose low glycaemic index (GI) carbohydrates — sweet potatoes, oats, wholegrain breads — (cut back on high GI carbohydrates — white breads, cakes, donuts, sugars etc).

  - Choose less sugar — RDA = 6 teaspoons (a western diet with processed foods can amount to 40 teaspoons a day)

- Essential fatty acids — choose more omega 3 (anti-inflammatory) — oily fish, walnuts, flax seeds, salmon, cherries, turmeric, dark green leafy vegetables, and soy. Choose less omega-6 and -9 (pro-inflammatory) — margarine, chips, cookies, cakes, biscuits, salad dressings, chocolate bars (although dark chocolate has natural antioxidant properties. Dark chocolate has also been shown to lower blood pressure — two squares after dinner only if it's 70 percent cocoa).

- Resveratol — found in skin of grapes, blueberries and raspberries, green tea. Have red wine with dinner (one or two glasses).

- Moderate use of yoghurt and low fat cheese

- Eat less meat and dairy

- If possible, all foods should be fresh, locally and organically grown.

- Electro-neuromodulation — this involves using electric current to modify pain perception. The most common and cheap method here is transcutaneous electrical nerve stimulation (TENS). TENS may work through these mechanisms

  - Prolonged stimulation causes the release of endorphins, resulting in a systemic analgesic effect.

  - Gate-close theory — afferent nerve pathways are blocked, limiting the transference of messages to the brain which are interpreted as pain. A more scientific explanation is that by stimulating the large A-beta mechanosensory fibres, nociceptor transmission is inhibited at the dorsal horn of the spinal cord (the brain doesn't receive the message clearly which can be interpreted as pain).

  - If the person is given control of the TENS unit, this may increase their perceived control of their pain, reducing the threat value and anxiety associated with the pain, thus modulating the pain experience.

- Other methods of electro-neuromodulation are high galvanic electrotherapy (mild electric impulse) and pulsed radiofrequency (PRF). PRF delivers an electromagnetic field, which modifies neuro-cellular function with minimal cellular destruction. These procedures have documented varying degrees of success (up to 80% for pelvic pain and urgency).

- InterX. The interX is an electrical device that provides interactive stimulation. The modality uses high amplitude, high density stimulation to the cutaneous nerves, activating the body's natural pain relieving mechanisms.

- Acupuncture, dry needling
- Pain Medication:
    - Simple analgesics — aspirin, paracetamol, tramadol
    - Anti-inflammatory drugs — NSAID
    - Pain Modulators — work on neurogenic pain — gabapentin, lyrica
    - Antidepressants — tricyclics and other groups
    - Narcotics — endone, oxycodeine + or - naloxone to prevent constipation, morphine.
- CT-guided pudendal nerve block techniques. There has been documentation of successful treatments by injecting the critical zone of compression of the pudendal nerve — mostly at the sacrospinous and sacrotuberous ligaments and the falciform process. The area is injected with lidocaine and long-release glucacorticoids.
- Botox injections into the suspected compressed areas.
- Myofascial Trigger Point releases and deep tissue massage. Myofascial Trigger Points are hyperirritable spots, usually within a taut band of skeletal muscle or the muscle's fascia. The spot is painful on compression and can give rise to a characteristic referred pain, tenderness and autonomic phenomenon. This spot can certainly contribute to the development of central sensitisation. Deep tissue massaging (and dry needling) has been found to be an effective treatment for reducing pain.

A Caution About Pain Management Treatments

I have a cautionary message to deliver when treating trigger points arising from an extremely oversensitive neuro-muscular system. I have found that by applying heavy palpatation, over-vigorous or prolonged treatments can re-trigger an already over-reactive neural system, creating an even more complex pain cycle. I personally don't apply trigger point massages or even deep tissue massages to any pudendal neuralgia patient, although I concede, with care (and experience), it may be a useful technique.

For the same reason, I am also very careful when prescribing pelvic floor exercises. The pudendal nerve supplies most of the pelvic floor muscles, which includes the urinary and anal sphincters. As these muscles (and sphincters) may also be in a chronic protective spasm cycle, (set off by any cause irritating the pudendal nerve) and be hypersensitive themselves, I have found aggressive pelvic floor exercises (and some other pelvic, abdominal, and low back exercises) can often trigger and maintain neural pain cycles. This is reinforced by Jerome Weiss's (2003) warning: any compression to an inflamed nerve (either by exercises or massage) not only can cause local pain, but also creates increased muscle tension which is transferred to the penetrating organs, i.e. the urethra, vagina, scrotum and rectum.

Finally, it is worthwhile reminding patients of this hopeful statement by Pearson (2007), who presents a well-formed explanation of the ability of patients with persistent pain to return to normal function:

> Remember, all these things that the nervous system has learned can be changed back. Neurons can become less sensitive; they can stop paying attention to and stop misinterpreting normal sensation as dangerous. Sensors can change back to the way they were; the map of the body on the brain can go back to its normal state and the muscles can regain their normal coordinated action. All it took was the wrong circumstances and lots of practice to get them to act the way they are. Now the patient has to practice new things. With Patience, Persistence, Compassion and Practice the patient will find ways to change them back, instead of just covering up the pain.

Chapter 4

Case Study Abstracts

A musculosketal approach for patients with pudendal neuralgia: A Cohort study

Published: British Journal of Urology International, November 2012

The objective of the study was to investigate the effect of musculoskeletal management of the lumbopelvic region in patients with pudendal neuralgia and musculoskeletal dysfunctions in the lumbopelvic region. Twenty-five patients with pudendal neuralgia without a nurological cause for the symptoms and with lumbopelvic musculoskeletal disorders participated. The intervention consisted of explanation and postural advice, specific manual mobilisation techniques and motor control exercises for the lumbopelvic region. A modified Pelvic Pain Symptom Survey was used to evaluate changes in pain and sexual dysfunction at the end of treatment and at three months follow-up. A repeated-measures analysis of variance was used to analyse the data. Results showed that at the end of the treatment period and at follow-up, pain and sexual dysfunction had improved significantly. Although 39% of patients had experienced limited recurrence of symptoms during the follow-up period, patients stated that a home exercise program was effective at reducing the symptoms and no additional treatment was sought. It was therefore concluded that this cohort study provides

Level 2b evidence that a musculoskeletal treatment approach has a positive influence on pain and sexual dysfunction in a specific subgroup of patients presenting with pudendal neuralgia

Faecal urgency and pelvic pain:
A case study implicating pudendal nerve entrapment

Published: Australian and New Zealand Continence Journal, Volume 18(1) 2012

The paper presents a case study describing the care of a man who presented with symptoms of faecal urgency and a diagnosis of sacroiliac joint dysfunction. The subject underwent six treatments over four weeks using manual mobilising techniques and motor control exercises. He reported lowered pain and urge levels. At 3 months follow-up the subject reported he was virtually symptom-free. The outcome suggests that, in some cases, faecel urgency may be a symptom of pudendal nerve entrapment and can be caused by sacroiliac joint dysfunction.

References

Introduction

Filler, A.G. (2009). Diagnosis and treatment of Pudendal Nerve Entrapment Syndromes Subtypes: Imaging, injections, and minimal access surgery. *Neurosurg Focus 26 (2):E92.*

Labat, J.J. et al. (1990). Journal d'Urologie 96 (5) 239-44.

Labat, J.J. et al. (2007). Neurology and Urodynamics. DOI 10.1002/nau

Mathias, S.D. et al. (1996). *Obstet Gynacol.* 87:321-327.

Prendergast, S.A., & Rummer, E.H., (2006). "The Role of Physical Therapy in Treatment of Pudendal Neuralgia". The International Pelvic Pain Society. *Vision.* Vol. 15. No. 1.

Roberts, R.D. et al. (1997). A review of clinical and pathological prostatitis syndrome. *Urology,* 49:809-821

Treede, R.D., Jensen, T.S. Campbell, J.N., Cruccu, G., Dostrovsky, J.O. et al. (2008). "Neuropathic pain. Redefinition and a grading system for clinical and research purposes". *Neurology,* April 29, Vol.70, No 18 1630-1635.

Weiss, J.M. 2003. Presented at the International Pelvic Pain Society, 10th Scientific meeting on Chronic Pelvic Pain in Alberta, Canada, August 2003.

Wise, D., & Anderson, R. 2008. *A Headache in the Pelvis.* 5th Edition 2008. Published by National Centre for Pelvic Pain Research. PO Box 54, Occidental Ca, 95465.

Chapter 1

Darnis, B., Robert, R., Labat, J.J., et al.(2008). Perineal pain and inferior cluneal nerves: Anatomy and surgery. *Surg Radiol Anat*. May; 30(3):177–83. Epub 2008 Feb 28

Jacob, H.A.C, Kissling, R.D. (1995). The mobility of the sacroiliac joints in healthy volunteers between 20 and 50 years of age, *Clin. Biomech*. (Bristol, Avon 10(7) 352

Lee, D. (2011). The Pelvic Girdle. Fourth Edition. P61. Elsevier.

Maigne, R. (1980). Low back pain of thorocolumbar origin. *Arch, Phys.Med*.Rehabil.61, 389–395

Maigne, R. (1981). Le Syndrome de la charmiere dorso-lombaire. Lombalgus basses, douleurs pseudo-viscerales, pseudo-douleurs de hanche, pseudo-tendinite des adducteurs. *Sem.Hop*. Paris. 57,11–12,545–554

Chapter 2

Hesch, J. (2011). Presented at the IPPS Workshop, Las Vegas.NV

Maitland, G.D. (2005). *Maitlands Vertebral Manipulation*, 7th ed. Philadelphia, PA. Elsevier.

Chapter 3

Computer Workstations: Design and adjustment. University of Queensland OHS. 2009

J. Hesch, J, (2011). Presented at the IPPS Workshop. Las Vegas NV.

Lee, D. (2011). *The Pelvic Girdle*. Fourth Edition. Elsevier.

Weiss, J.M. (2003). presented at the International pelvic Pain Society 10th Scientific Meeting, on Chronic Pelvic Pain in Alberta, Canada.

Pearson, N. (2007). *Understand Pain, Live Well Again*. Penticton, British Columbia, Canada, Life is Now.

Further Reading

Explain Pain, David Butler and Lorimer Mosely. Norgroup Publications, Adelaide. S.Australia. (August 2010 Reprint)

Heal Pelvic Pain. Amy Stein. McGraw Hill. New York. 2009

CPSIA information can be obtained at www.ICGtesting.com
Printed in the USA
LVOW09s1542110615

442114LV00007B/144/P